CRYING IN
CUPBOARDS

PTo

CRYING IN CUPBOARDS

WHAT HAPPENS WHEN TEACHERS ARE BULLIED?

Pat Bricheno and Mary Thornton

Matador
9 Priory Business Park,
Wistow Road, Kibworth Beauchamp,
Leicestershire. LE8 0RX
Tel: 0116 279 2299
Email: books@troubador.co.uk
Web: www.troubador.co.uk/matador
Twitter: @matadorbooks

ISBN 978 1785892 752

British Library Cataloguing in Publication Data.
A catalogue record for this book is available from the British Library.

Printed and bound by CPI Group (UK) Ltd, Croydon, CR0 4YY
Typeset in 11pt Minion Pro by Troubador Publishing Ltd, Leicester, UK

Matador is an imprint of Troubador Publishing Ltd

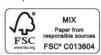

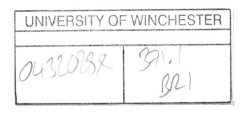

Contents

SECTION TWO: WHAT THE TEACHERS, MANAGERS
AND UNIONS SAID

SECTION THREE: WHAT WE KNOW ABOUT THE BULLYING OF
TEACHERS NOW

Acknowledgements

Many people have helped us in our research for this book. Our special thanks go to all those teachers who volunteered their stories, and were prepared to speak freely to us about the highly emotional and harmful experience of being bullied in both their professional lives and their specific work places.

When we first interviewed these teachers, many were ill, and some were very ill indeed. The interview sessions proved to be distressing, on both sides. Nevertheless, it has been a pleasure and a privilege to hear of the recovery and progress that so many of our teacher volunteers have made over the past three years.

We would also like to thank all the Headteachers, Deputy Heads and Union officials who gave willingly of their time, advice and insights regarding our particular teachers' experiences of being bullied in schools, and their combined wisdom regarding how such issues might best be addressed. We are particularly grateful to union representatives from the Association of Teachers and Lecturers, the National Association of Schoolmasters/Union of Women Teachers and the National Union of Teachers amongst others for their assistance with this project.

Our thanks go to the Education Support Partnership (formerly TSN), a long term trusted supporter, who helped and encouraged us along the way and who provided us with the means to find our volunteer teachers.

Finally we thank our families and friends who have supported and encouraged us during the course of this work. We are especially grateful to Lyanne Thornton-Harewood for both assisting with the transcriptions and designing and producing the cover photo and to Robert Bricheno for the cover design.

We trust that our readers and supporters find these endeavours to have been worthwhile.

Preface

A great deal has been written about children being bullied, both in schools and on the internet, and there is emerging research on the cyber-bullying of teachers by some parents. However, little is known, or heard, about teachers being bullied by the adults that they work with inside their schools. Most schools have their own specific policies and procedures for dealing with different issues and behaviours, many mandated from above. Schools are rule governed organisations that invariably present themselves, to their local community and the wider world, as being safe, caring and harmonious places in which to work and study. But in some schools this aspirational public face masks a somewhat more hidden world of oppressive accountability and grading, increasing pressure and decreasing job security; resulting in heightened stress levels, anxiety and potential depression. Such schools are considerably less safe, caring and harmonious environments in which to work than their public face might usually suggest. This book seeks to shed light on this somewhat more hidden world through its exploration of teachers' experiences of being bullied.

We wrote this book mainly for the teachers themselves, for their stories to be heard, and so that the problem of teachers being bullied might be more widely recognised and potentially addressed. We hope that the exploration and identification of factors that might contribute to the problem or aggravate its occurrence will be useful to school managers, union officials and policy makers too. The 'churn' of teachers, including their potential departure from the profession, is exacerbated by the bullying that takes place. But it is rarely named as such because more acceptable labels are preferred and negotiated, in order to maintain good references and a career, to facilitate moving on, or to avoid the additional stresses imposed by often unwinnable conflicts and official tribunals.

We have tried hard to write in a way that makes the book as accessible to the general public and non-expert reader as it is to the much smaller academic and research community that would usually be the main audience for such evidence-based work. With these different audiences in mind we have divided the book into sections that can be dipped into in any order depending on the needs and interests of the reader.

Section 1: 'What we already know about bullying' seeks primarily to address the issues and to answer questions that would normally concern the academic and research communities. The three chapters in this section directly address the historical and organisational context (Chapter 1), the extant literature (Chapter 2) and the research methods employed, together with a brief but more traditional presentation of the data and findings (Chapter 3).

Section 2: 'What the teachers, senior school managers and teacher unions said' (about bullying) is the real heart of this book. This is the section that general readers may well read first. It is here that we give greater voice to the real-life experiences of bullying in schools encountered by teachers, Senior Managers and Union officials. Section 2 begins with the teachers' stories about being bullied (Chapter 4). In order to maintain the essential and promised confidentiality regarding each individual's unique experiences (and their school's identity), the accounts are presented as stories. This is followed by detailed responses and commentaries about our teachers' experiences from Senior Managers, mostly Headteachers (Chapter 5) and Union officials

(Chapter 6), together with more general observations based on their knowledge and understanding of the problem.

Section 3: 'What we know about the bullying of teachers now' revisits the literature on bullying that is explored in section 1, and draws some conclusions based on our research (Chapter 7). Finally, Chapter 8 offers a brief 'two years on' update on what has happened to our bullied teachers since they first told us about their experiences.

Most are now in a better place but, as the reader will see, the scars will likely remain.

SECTION ONE

What we already know about bullying

Introduction

Section one sets the scene for our research, examining what is already known about workplace bullying. The academic and research community will likely be the main audience for this articulation of evidence-based work, but those who choose to read Sections 2 and 3 first might well want to dip into it later. In Chapter 1 we describe the context within which our research is located. First the particular historical context; that of the UK, and primarily English, education system in the years following the 1988 Education Reform Act (ERA: DES, 1988), and then the sociological and organisational context.

Next, in Chapter 2, we review the existing research that is related to workplace bullying, focusing first on individual characteristics such as age, gender, ethnicity and disability. We then discuss the research concerning work environment and organisation; looking at how demand, control, support, power, organisational changes and leadership styles relate to workplace bullying.

Our own research is described in Chapter 3 beginning with our volunteers: who they were, how we found them and how we interviewed them. We then give a brief overview of our findings: what the teachers described to us, who they said was responsible for their bullying, the environments in which they worked, the support they received and the impact the bullying had on them. We move on to describe the reasons offered by the teachers, by Senior Managers in schools and by Union officials for the bullying, finishing with a consideration of the ways forward suggested by these three groups.

1

CONTEXT

1.1

Historical and Organisational Context

The 1988 Education Reform Act (DES, 1988), enacted more than 25years ago, is pivotal to our understanding of the structures and context in which teachers today are reporting increasing levels of stress and bullying behaviour in schools. Since then education and teaching in England has changed profoundly, with relocated and reallocated formal positions of power, new opportunities for the exercise of informal power, and the creation of immense pressures and strains upon teachers and school leaders through constant change and ever increasing monitoring of their performance for accountability purposes.

Teachers are not an homogenous group of people; there is great variety amongst them as well as great diversity in how they respond to changes in their work environments. However, those who trained to teach before 1988 would now be in their late 40's at least, potentially the Headteachers or senior staff in schools, while their youngest of colleagues will remember nothing of pre-ERA schools beyond, perhaps, their own experience as pupils, and they will have trained to teach post-ERA, albeit with possibly lingering alternative philosophies within their teacher training experience from a different, pre-ERA landscape.

Understanding the importance of the ERA requires us to go back even further in time, to when the Plowden Report (DES, 1967) noted that teachers who advise and inspire, rather than instruct, were at the forefront of a new and developing child-centred educational philosophy, a development that the report recommended should extend beyond the Primary school, into the early Secondary school years. Alongside Plowden's focus on a child-centred approach there was a wider view of teachers as professionals, engaged in collegial or collaborative activities that fostered development and learning in their pupils. Whilst traditional subjects were taught and exams prepared for in Secondary schools, teachers and schools, under the guidance of their Local Authorities (LAs)[1] were largely left to determine what was taught, when and to whom, primarily on the basis of teachers' professional judgement.

The publication of the Plowden Report was a context changing event that marked the end of education's 40 years of freedom from statutory government control and direct political intervention in the pedagogy teachers adopted and the curriculum they delivered. Multiple reports on education followed, and it became increasingly clear that government, regardless of its political orientation, officially ceased to be neutral or 'hands off' regarding education. Until 1982 teachers had control of the school curriculum, albeit at times constrained by the 11+ and later by secondary examination systems. That 'Secret Garden' (Lawton, 1973) gradually fell under direct political control. Between 1983 and 1987 there were 15 major reports or initiatives (averaging 3 a year), some covering teacher training, and culminating in 'The National Curriculum 5-16: A consultative document' (1987), which was followed by something of a tidal wave of official documents after the 1988 Education Reform Act (ERA) came into effect.

The ERA 1988 was essentially a Standards agenda (Evans, 2011) enshrined in statute. The National Curriculum 5-16 specified the curriculum subjects and the subject specific content that had to be taught in all English and Welsh schools.

---

1   Previously referred to as LEAs

It came with compulsory annual testing (Standardized Assessment Tasks, SATs) for children aged 7, 11 and 14 years, and was followed by the publication of school league tables based on raw SATs data (Troman, 2008).The notion of value-added league tables came later, as did the specification and subsequent inflation of minimum percentage passes at GCSE of A* to C grades. Importantly, the ERA allowed schools to become independent of their LAs either by becoming funded directly by central government (City Technology Colleges and Grant Maintained Schools), or by adopting Local Management of Schools (LMS), both of which placed direct financial control in the hands of Headteachers and their school governing bodies. The principle of school choice was also introduced in the 1988 Act, whereby parents could specify which school was their preferred choice, with parental decisions made often on the basis of position in the school league tables.

Schools directly funded by government and those administered under LMS both brought work insecurity to teachers in a form not previously experienced, except perhaps in the Victorian days, of 'payment by results':

> 'Previously teacher salaries were paid for by the LEA and teaching posts were safeguarded by a regional commitment to job security so that teachers who were surplus to one school's requirements would be redeployed in another school. The change in the law has meant that each teacher's job security is restricted to their employability within one school. Furthermore, that employability is linked to the success of the school to attract sufficient numbers of pupils to guarantee the teacher's wages'.

> (Humphreys, 1994: 189)

Work security for teachers in England[2] is now firmly dependent upon individual school finances, the Headteacher and the school governing body. Finances in turn depend on a school's success in the educational market place of Ofsted (Office for Standards in Education) inspections, public accountability, league table position and parental choice. Individual job security is also now dependent upon assessments made of the teacher's work by Ofsted and local managers, most usually the Headteacher, who guides and advises their governing body about staffing, and who is able to make powerful recommendations regarding an individual's fitness to teach (Capability) and continued employment within the school. Thus, formal power over teachers' work and employment is now vested in school managers, most usually the Headteacher, without the more distanced oversight and perspectives of LAs and former inspectors of schools (HMI) being brought to bear. LMS and the limitation of LA oversight and direct control, alongside ever greater powers and responsibilities residing with Headteachers left teachers '...*very wary about being critical of their controlling superiors. This is especially the case when LMS is leading to many schools having to lose staff...*' (Humphreys, 1994: 187)

School Development Plans (SDPs), part of the LMS imperative, contributed to teachers' ever increasing workloads (Gu & Day, 2013; Addison & Brundrett, 2008), with Webb and Vulliamy, citing Ball (1984: 61), arguing that the '*SDP signifies and celebrates the exclusion and subjection of the teacher. Not only does the teacher lose control over classroom planning decisions, but will be monitored, judged and compared by criteria set elsewhere.*'(Webb & Vulliamy, 1996: 452)

The 1990s saw many special needs pupils integrated into mainstream schooling, which required teachers to produce

---

2   Unless otherwise stated the national context being referred to throughout is that of England

personal development plans for them, and later individualised learning plans for all. In recognition of ever increasing workloads a Planning and Preparation Allowance (PPA) was introduced, alongside cover for qualified teachers provided by a new stratum of school employee, the classroom teacher assistant or TA, whose work had to be designed, assigned and monitored by the very teachers they were employed to help and relieve of some aspects of their workload (Addison & Brundrett, 2008; Troman, 2008).

The role, responsibilities and constitution of school governing bodies also changed significantly post ERA and LMS. There is now far greater diversity between school types and funding regimes, and their respective degrees of autonomy. This impacts on the nature of and style in which schools are governed, but they all continue to operate under the oversight of governing bodies. While LA input is seriously eroded and continuing to decline, governing bodies are now expected to be representative of 'stakeholders' in the school system. This would usually include parents and staff (elected members) and community, and local business (co-opted members).

The main school governor roles are oversight, monitoring, challenging and supporting the school, its staff, pupils and their academic outcomes (Dean, Dyson, Gallannaugh, Howes & Raffo, 2007; National Governors' Association website, 2015). James, Brammer, Connoly, Spicer, James & Jones, (2013) suggest that, from their research, scrutiny rather than critical friendship or challenge is now the preferred modus operandi of school governors, while Dean et al., (2007:ix) suggest that governors feel happier offering support rather than challenges to their schools and staffs. However, increasingly the focus for governors has been on holding the Headteacher and senior management team to account, managing performance – including that of the Headteacher, *ensuring financial probity and appropriate use of resources, alongside encouraging parental involvement and ensuring pupil safety'* (James et al.,2013: 85). The focus on financial probity and school management is increasingly a concern for governing bodies now that funding is largely devolved to schools (Earley et al., 2012). Interesting, the large scale survey of leadership personnel in schools conducted by Earley et al., makes no mention of governors' roles in staff appraisal, discipline or Capability Proceedings (CPs) when reporting the responses of the chairs of school governing bodies to their questions about school leadership. It may be because they were not asked the appropriate questions but, in terms of Chair of Governors' main reported activities' there is no mention of these aspects of their work, and this absence from such a recent large-scale and well-funded report is significant in terms of understanding teacher stress and reports of bullying.

With the advent of Free Schools under the Conservative coalition (2010-15) the complexity and diversity amongst schools and their governance has been further increased: put simply, schools have become *'more complex to lead and to manage, especially in terms of budgets, human resources, professional development and administration...'* (Earley et al., 2012: viii).

School governors are, in effect and in law, *'...line managers between the school and the Secretary of State.'* (Humphreys, 1994: 190). At the same time their effectiveness in fulfilling their increased responsibilities has been called into question. Ofsted (2012) now includes school governance in its inspection criteria, and governing bodies can be both suspended or replaced depending on inspection outcomes. Many governing bodies are found to be fundamentally supportive of their Headteacher (Dean et al., 2007: 37) and readily endorse Heads' recommendations or decisions, rather than fully exercising their designated role as a 'critical friend' (Earley, et al., 2012), or their legal position as the body to whom teachers can appeal if they believe they have been unfairly treated.

The post–ERA centrally-prescribed curriculum and pedagogy resulted in a shift away from reliance on teachers' professional skills and knowledge towards a much more prescriptive approach to teaching, where teachers are expected to deliver pre-specified content in recommended ways, sometimes referred to as a 'technicist' approach. Conformity to these prescriptions is measured at every turn, from Ofsted inspection, through performance review and annual appraisal to Performance Related Pay (PRP).

At the same time top-down accountability, quality assurance and a Standards agenda was being led by Ofsted. Ofsted was established in 1992 and its main purpose was to collect evidence to set against statutory criteria, and to make public their resulting assessments. Ofsted inspections are incredibly important for schools and teachers: their outcomes affect funding (through league tables and parental choice), status, careers and job security (failing schools may be closed, weak ones placed in special measures, and teaching careers terminated). It is inevitable that teachers and schools pay close attention to Ofsted's inspection criteria. Checklists and 'guides to inspection' are readily available and widely used, supporting a technicist 'painting by numbers' approach (Humphreys, 1994:181) to inspection. Case, Case and Catling, (2000) describe this as the stage-managing of their performance whilst under Ofsted's glare. However, curriculum guides and pedagogic checklists extend well beyond Ofsted inspections, and appear to be widely used. There can be no doubt that a great many teachers (and Heads) feel 'professionally compromised, intimidated and stressed by the inspection process' (Case, Case & Catling, 2000: 605), and that inspections have contributed significantly to the increase in technicist approaches to teaching, both during and beyond the inspection process.

Statutory measures of teacher performance have always been part of Ofsted inspections, and the enormity of the impact of Ofsted judgements has brought with it high levels of anxiety and stress amongst teachers, not least because they have also led to increased monitoring activity of teacher performance by Heads and other managers/ school leaders. In 1996 Webb and Vulliamy argued that the inspection process and its requirements *'...was leading Headteachers to operate as resident inspectors in order to monitor the classroom performance of their teachers...',* and that this climate of inspection encouraged *'...Headteachers to be powerful and, if necessary, manipulative leaders...'* (Webb & Vulliamy, 1996: 448). Whilst Ofsted inspections come and go the monitoring and assessment of teacher performance and effectiveness locally, by Heads and line managers, is now constant and ubiquitous.

Professional Standards were formally introduced into schools in September 2007, and refer to teacher appraisal against agreed and established standards of teaching (Evans, 2011). What is most important about the specification and delineation of Professional Standards for teachers is the 'performative' aspect that describes them, and this links back, directly, to the technicist approach to teaching that has accompanied post-ERA reforms. Citing Beck (2009: 8), Evans argues that the standards discourse *'...suggests that being a professional educator is a matter of acquiring a limited corpus of state prescribed knowledge accompanied by a set of similarly prescribed skills and competencies. The model is a technicist one involving the acquisition of trainable expertise'* (Evans, 2011: 861).

Our teacher interviews were conducted in 2012. It was a busy period in terms of public statements about education and teachers, many of which added to the pressure and scrutiny that teachers were under. For example, in September 2011 Michael Gove, then Secretary of State for Education, questioned why some schools were rated 'outstanding' by Ofsted when the learning and teaching within them wasn't also graded at this level; in December 2011 Sir Michael Wilshaw, then Head-designate of

Ofsted stated that, '*If anyone says to you that 'staff morale is at an all-time low' you will know you are doing something right*', and he promised to bring PRP into the classroom, together with an inspection focus on teacher '*dress and demeanour*'. In May 2012 he proclaimed that '*teachers are not stressed*' whilst promising that the climate for Ofsted inspections would be '*unforgiving*', with schools given just 1 days notice (later overruled by Michael Gove). As a result Wilshaw was himself accused of bullying behaviour at the 2012 National Association of Head Teachers (NAHT) Conference. In August 2012 he noted that a third of schools were 'not good' (i.e. they were merely satisfactory); in September 2012 the inspection categories that Gove had questioned were changed: 'satisfactory' was discontinued and all schools are now required to achieve an Ofsted rating of 'good' or better by 2016.

PRP was introduced in 2014, along with annual appraisal in school and locally determined pay scales. A very close link has been established between teacher pay and performance, as decided and judged internally by schools, their managers and governors. The government's aim, they claim, isn't necessarily to cut the pay of hard-working teachers, but to create a stronger link between pay and performance, with each school now required to make clear specific links between proposed future teacher pay and their past assessed classroom performances (DfE, 2013). Taking LMS to its ultimate extreme individual schools (and their Heads/managers and governing bodies) are now required to assess teachers' individual teaching standards, and their pupils' achievements, against government determined criteria, and decide on that basis any possible pay increase. Mandatory pay points have been abolished and individual schools given the freedom to decide how much their teachers are paid.

Many new management roles, responsibilities and structures have been created post-ERA, from new subject leader and examination co-ordination roles in Primary schools to assistant Heads working alongside Heads, their Deputies and senior administrators or bursars in Secondary schools, in order to meet the ever increasing demands for documentation and devolved financial responsibilities. There are many more people holding junior and senior management roles in schools now than there were before the reforms, and these people are themselves held accountable through monitoring, appraisal and school inspections for the delivery of those reforms and the latest government policy initiatives. There is tremendous pressure on all staff in schools to meet the targets set for them, and the growth in managerialism (Troman & Woods, 2001) can be seen as one mechanism that works to achieve that.

So where does this historical overview and contextualisation of teachers' work in compulsory education in England lead us? Primarily it leads us to a recognition of the unremitting pressures, stresses and strains that have become core features of teachers' current and ongoing working lives, the prescriptive environments in which they work, and their increasingly fragile career security. There can be no doubt that the English education system *'has undergone a series of rapid, multiple and systemic changes since the 1988 Education Act which are likely to have affected teachers' motivation and morale.'* (Addison & Brundrett, 2008: 79)

To be strong and to survive in this current pressure-cooker environment teachers need positive encouragement, praise, and Headteacher/manager support, what Gu and Day refer to as leadership support and, *'the ability of the principals to buffer the effects of external changes'* (2013: 38). Such support is critical to teachers' commitment, performance and career survival. However, there are many de-motivators, such as workload, ever changing directives and targets, constant observation and performance monitoring, and these may well be the cause of the stresses and strains that teachers report. Performativity pressures, external accountability and work complexity (Gu &

Day, 2013: 40) effectively work to debilitate teachers (Troman, 2008). Failures to meet their allotted targets or to perform adequately are key contributors to teacher stress, and are linked to bullying behaviour.

Accountability control structures are now both internal to schools (pay, appraisal, performance management, and continual monitoring and assessment by school Heads/managers), and external, most notably in the league tables of test results, in public GCSE and A level examination results, and of course Ofsted inspections, which publicly hold teachers and their schools to account; these underpin and support both hierarchies and markets in education (West, Mattel & Roberts, 2011: 41). We would argue that the newly established internal control structures, alongside the external climate of inspection may well have had a significant impact in terms of the incidence and veracity of teachers' reports of bullying in schools.

With such pressures on Heads and senior school management, as well as on junior managers and classroom teachers, there is greater opportunity and possibly also greater reason for the newly defined and acquired formal and informal positions of power within schools to be used (enacted) and potentially abused, resulting in bullying behaviours.

Troman and Wood argued (2001) that the intensification of teachers' work, as outlined above, has led not only to increased stress but also to the reconstruction of their individual identities as teachers. For Troman (2008: 630), *'the holism, humanism and vocationalism of the old Plowden self-identity has been challenged by a new, assigned social identity...'* while Ball notes (2003: 215) that *'it changes who they are'*. Teachers' sense of self, their social identity, has undoubtedly been reshaped by and through the reforms of the past 25 years, as have the varied locations of formal (and informal) power resources in schools, along with the ability of many different actors to activate them.

Sociological Explanations of Workplace Bullying

Most sociological explorations of bullying in the workplace are in essence 'grand narratives' about capital and labour in conflict (Roscigno, Lopez & Hodson, 2009). The focus is primarily on industrial relations and the extent of unionisation in large organisations with many layers of junior and senior managers and workers, most particularly at times of change in terms of restructuring or downsizing (Beale & Hoel, 2011; Ferris, Zinko, Brouer, Buckley & Harvey, 2007). In such places people can become victims of bullying at the hands of seniors while at the same time being bullies themselves towards those beneath them, often in pursuit of personal and organisational goals. Beale and Hoel (2011) suggest that this can lead to possible gains for organisations, for example in terms of targets, outputs and profits that can be set against the potential costs of bullying in terms of staff turnover, tribunals and sick leave. Lowly placed, unskilled workers with little autonomy are most frequently found to be victims of bullying (Ferris et al., 2007) whilst skilled workers with valued knowledge, working independently in a *professional and collegial environment* are likely to be less vulnerable to bullying behaviours (Roscigno, Hodson & Lopez, 2009: 755).

Despite the dramatic shift away from the autonomous professional and collegial working of schools and teachers post-ERA, and the substantial evidence of a profession under extreme stress and strain from intrusive and severe accountability procedures, in *relative* terms and in relation to other workers, teachers remain highly skilled, well-paid, and independent, working in professional teams in what it is usually characterised as a collegial working environment where people and values matter.

In their extensive study of 'Trouble at Work', Fevre, et al., (2012) use a sociological approach to explore and measure the characteristics of organisational culture in different workplaces as these move '*from collective to individualised employment relations*' (p.226). As sociologists they are particularly interested in structural conflicts that take place in capitalist workplaces, between employers and employees, where bullying is endemic and primarily used by employers and managers to change employee behaviour. Their work was predicated on the view that troubled workplaces would be places where '*individuals did not matter*', and this led them to rely heavily on interviewees responses to three specific statements that they used to identify particularly troubled workplaces. The specific statements are (p.52):

- Where I work, the needs of the organisation always come before the needs of people
- Where I work, you have to compromise your principles
- Where I work, people are not treated as individuals

While Fevre et al., identify many troubled workplaces using this approach, they found that workers in education are among the least likely to agree with those three statements – about having to compromise their principles, about not being treated as an individual, and especially about the needs of the organisation coming first, before people. This leads them to suggest that education might be an exceptional case, where perhaps more individual or psychological explanations of bullying might apply. This may or may not be the case. However, their premise that *individuals did not matter*, and their over-reliance on responses to specific questionnaire statements that might demonstrate it, had the effect of excluding teachers and schools from their sociological analysis of 'trouble at work', despite the high incidence of reported 'trouble' in school workplaces. It is also clear that bullying or 'trouble' in schools does not fit well within their industrial relations/ sociological model of bullying.

Most ill-treatment (or bullying) of workers is done by their managers. Fevre et al., interpret this as employer-employee conflict around '*authority and control rather than power distance*' (p.201). However, in school workplaces direct organisational conflicts such as these appear to be rare. In schools, teachers will more usually experience persistent ill-treatment and undermining based on the abuse or misuse of power. As such teacher bullying appears to relate more closely to power disparity and people than it does to organisational structures and conflicts.

The possession, exercise and direction of power within education and schools might also be a contributory factor to the 'exceptionality' of education as a 'troubled' workplace.

Following Foucault (2002, 1998), we see power as something that is fluid rather than fixed, multi-directional and mobile, originating in the discourses that surround and encompass us all and which shape our individual sense of ourselves. Using a Foucauldian perspective, Fahie and Devine (2012: 5) argue that power is based in and on our relationships with others, and is exercised in complex ways within bullying relationships, with the victim subject to losing their sense of self as a teacher or professional. Their study of Irish teachers who reported being bullied suggests that not only were the teachers' professional careers compromised but that many actually resigned from their internally promoted posts, left teaching altogether, or took early retirement or alternative employment instead. As Foucault might have predicted, their sense of self/ self-identity had been reshaped by the bullying discourse within which they found themselves. For Fahie and Devine (2012: 10), '...*the bullying discourse subjectifies these teachers as ineffective and, in some way, 'deserving' of the negative behaviours'*, and *'arises from attempts to 'subject' and control the actions and identity of the victim...'*, fundamentally changing how the victims sees themselves. In teaching as in other workplaces, micro-management or excessive supervision can undermine autonomy and remove control over one's work, and may be a particularly powerful form of bullying because it increases feelings of powerlessness on the part of victims (Vartia, 1996). In part this might explain the apparent lack of collective action against bullying behaviours.

Power, in the Foucauldian sense, is something that is exercised rather than held. The capacity to exclude, demean, abuse, harass, undermine, slander or threaten – all reported types of bullying behaviours – is present in many if not most of our lived social contexts and relationships and in the discourses of our workplaces, but it is not the same thing as its enactment – power is located in the realisation of that capacity. Power can be exercised formally on the basis of hierarchy, position or status, but it can also be exercised informally, for example on the basis of contacts with influential people or individual standing; through experience, knowledge and/ or access to social support (Einarsen, Hoel & Notelaers, 2009); or having knowledge of others vulnerabilities (Hoel & Cooper 2001; Rayner, Hoel & Cooper, 2002).

Sociological theories of workplace bullying do articulate with some of the views of the Union officials that we interviewed, particularly in terms of seeking collective responses to bullies and bullying behaviours. However, we found most self-reporting of bullying by victims was primarily an individual rather than a group response, although sometimes there was more than one victim in a particular school. There was also a lack of overt peer support for bullied colleagues, and a great deal of fear about reprisals and/or becoming the next target for the bully. As a largely individualised experience of the enactment of power, teacher bullying appears less amenable to collective solutions than sociological theory or Union officials might suggest, despite strong union membership and well established collective action regarding teacher pay or conditions.

2

THE LITERATURE

2.1

Background

Although many definitions of workplace bullying are found in the literature, there is a general consensus regarding what constitutes bullying (Einarsen, Hoel, Zapf & Cooper, 2003). Frequency, imbalance of power and repeated behaviours are mentioned in the majority of definitions '... *repeated and persistent negative acts towards one or more individual(s), which involve a perceived power imbalance and create a hostile work environment*' (Salin, 2003:4). Major teacher unions in the United Kingdom share a similar definition of bullying in the educational workplace, regarding it as '...*the persistent (and normally deliberate) misuse of power or position to intimidate, humiliate or undermine*' (NUT, NASUWT, ATL)[3]. Our definition of bullying uses Salin's general definition in combination with the specific behaviours indicated by the main UK teaching unions that are consistent with those from the research literature.

Internationally there are different labels for bullying but also some agreement over what constitutes bullying (above), and there are consistencies within the behaviours identified, such as persistent insults, criticism or ridicule (e.g. Hoel & Cooper, 2000; Leymann, 1996), being ignored or treated as non-existent (e.g. Einarsen & Raknes, 1997; Rayner & Hoel, 1997), given demeaning tasks or set up to fail (Bentley et al., 2009; Rayner &

---

3   NUT= National Union of Teachers; NASUWT=National Association of Schoolmasters and Women Teachers; ATL= Association of Teachers and Lecturers

Hoel, 1997), arbitrary removal of responsibilities or being given unrealistic work demands (Lewis & Gunn, 2007; Einarsen & Raknes, 1997). Within these behaviours, Einarsen et al., (2003) note that some are personal in origin (name calling, teasing, insulting) while others are organisationally derived (increasing workloads, excessive performance monitoring).

In a formal sense the power structures of schools, as organisations, can in part explain the large number of teachers who report that they are being bullied by their Headteacher or Senior Managers. It is the role of senior staff to manage and make judgements about those beneath them, and on some occasions, in some instances, it is possible that such legitimate actions are perceived as bullying by those on the receiving end.

Importantly, reports of bullying in schools are not limited to, or fully explained by, formal hierarchical power imbalance: for example, in an NASUWT survey (2011) 20% of teachers named others, including Admin/Support staff, main scale co-teachers or classroom teaching assistants (TAs) as the bully, and the folklore that abounds around the informal power exercised by caretakers (janitors) and classroom cleaners is unlikely to be completely without foundation: *'The abuse of informal power can be enacted by workers in any position (e.g. spreading rumours) against targets in any position... It should be noted that workers with formal power also have informal power'* (McGrath, 2010:3). It is the perceived or actual misuse/ abuse of that power imbalance that is the principal problem in teacher-reported bullying, not imbalance per se.

In earlier research (Thornton & Bricheno, 2006) we invited teachers who were leaving, or had already left, the profession to tell us their reasons for leaving. Nine percent of the 371 respondents said they were leaving, or had left, because of bullying, usually by someone more senior than themselves. Many linked being bullied with lack of support from colleagues, senior management or governors, and with health issues, in particular stress-related illness and depression, and most gave brief outlines of the mistreatment they had suffered at work, including unrealistic expectations, high workloads, lack of trust and constant change (Bricheno & Thornton, 2006). That earlier research is supported by a number of other studies that also find that workplace bullying is associated with leaving or intention to leave: some of it with teachers (McCormack, Casimir, Djurkovic & Yang, 2009; Blasé, Blasé & Du, 2008; Djurkovic, McCormack & Casimir, 2008) and some relating to other workers (Fetherston & Lummis, 2012; Berthelsen, Skogstad, Lau & Einarsen, 2011: Bentley et al., 2009; Quine, 2001). In our earlier research (cited above) some teachers gave detailed descriptions of their mistreatment. For example:

'I was recently bullied by my Headteacher, and was suspended over fictitious allegations. In spite of the fact I was reinstated without any sort of reprimand, my Headteacher refused to accept it, and has made my life hell. It is a hard enough job anyway but this made it worse and affected my health. Had I stayed I am in no doubt I would have had a complete nervous breakdown. My Headteacher has since harassed and bullied at least 4 other staff, all of whom have left the school in similar circumstances to me. The rest of the staff are still suffering. There seems to be very little we can do to stop this woman, even though she has a record of similar behaviour in her previous school. The governors have been completely unsupportive and couldn't care less'.

Such comments give us a small taste of what might be described as bullying by some teachers, but what does the literature have to say about what counts as workplace bullying?

Research into work-place bullying, which originated as a concept in Scandinavian countries, emerged as a subject of world-wide interest during the 1990s. A very large body of work now exists on the subject of workplace bullying and yet, as Fevre et al.,(2012) point out, it remains difficult '*to decide what counts as bullying at work*', that there is '*far too much inconsistency in the application of the label of bullying*'. They contend that '*the bullying label is not sufficiently familiar to, and similarly understood by, British employees to allow a general explanation*' (Fevre et al., 2012: 28).

Whilst '*bullying*' is the term most frequently used in the UK and Australia, this behaviour is generally referred to as '*mobbing*' in Scandinavian and German speaking countries (Einarsen, Hoel, Zapf & Cooper, 2011; Di Martino Hoel & Cooper, 2003). In the USA similar phenomena have been given a wide variety of labels, including '*workplace harassment*', '*mistreatment*' and, more recently, '*employee abuse*' and '*workplace aggression*' (Keashly & Jagatic, 2011). However, Einarsen et al., (2011: 31) maintain that despite their cultural diversity and the use of different terms Europeans have '*largely succeeded in developing and maintaining a shared conceptual understanding of the underlying phenomenon*' of workplace bullying.

Surveys aimed at measuring the prevalence of bullying that occurs in the workplace have generated data from a diversity of countries and cultures (for example, China: Turkey, Australia, UK, and the USA) and via a wide range of methods; some, referred to as 'self-labelling', ask simply whether or not respondents believe they have been bullied, some also provide a definition of what the researchers regard as bullying behaviour, although many do not. Usually respondents will also be asked how often the bullying occurs and who the perpetrator is. Other surveys ask a series of behavioural questions without reference to the word bullying, usually in conjunction with a later question asking about bullying at work, accompanied by a definition of workplace bullying. A well validated and reliable behavioural questionnaire is the Negative Acts Questionnaire (Hoel, Rayner

& Cooper, 1999; Einarsen, Raknes & Matthiesen, 1994) in which all items are written in behavioural terms with no reference to the terms 'bullying' or 'harassment'. Examples include[4]:

- Being ignored or excluded.
- Having allegations made against you.
- Being exposed to an unmanageable workload.
- Excessive monitoring of your work.
- Being shouted at or being the target of spontaneous anger.

After responding to these items, a definition of bullying at work is given and participants are asked to indicate whether or not they consider themselves as victims according to the definition.

A comparison of these different approaches, using a meta-analysis of 102 prevalence studies, provides some useful average figures (Neilsen, Matthiesen & Einarsen, 2010). The average values quoted for the prevalence of workplace bullying are as follows:

- Self-labelling based on a given definition 11.3%.
- Behavioural measures 14.8%.
- Self-labelling without a given definition 18.1%.

Because of the large difference found between self-labelling with or without a definition Neilsen, Matthiesen & Einarsen, (2010) suggest that participants in research studies may not understand the bullying concept in the same way as the researchers and therefore, they recommend, future self-labelling studies should include a definition.

Zapf, Escartin, Einarsen, Hoel & Vartia (2011) reviewing bullying studies across all types of measurement and sampling, looked at the criterion of the frequency of bullying and suggest

---

4   For a more extensive list see Appendix

that severe bullying (at least once a week) probably occurs for between 3% and 4%, but with a less strict criterion of bullying (less than once a week) the estimate rises to between 10% and 15%. In addition, where no definition is provided and self-labelling is used the figure rises to 20% (Neilsen, Skogstad, Matthiesen, Glasø, Aasland, Notelaers & Einarsen, 2009).

Such widely differing prevalence values leads us to question how much workplace bullying of teachers really occurs in schools. According to the fourth European Working Survey (Parent-Thirion, Macías, Hurley & Vermeylen, 2007) the risk of experiencing bullying and harassment is greatest in the education and health sectors. Other studies, for example Hubert and Veldhoven (2001) and Zapf et al., (2011), report similar data on the incidence of bullying in these sectors. Over time, a diverse range of statistical studies aimed at measuring the prevalence of workplace bullying specifically among teachers have emerged, including, for example, those listed in Table 1 below.

Table 1: Examples of the prevalence (%) of workplace bullying of teachers

Country	Authors	Sample	Measure Used	%
Ireland	INTO* (2000)	402	Behavioural	36
Turkey	Cemaloglu (2007)#	337	Behavioural	6.4
Croatia	Russo et al.,(2008)	764	Behavioural	22.4
New Zealand	Bentley et al.,(2009)	459	Behavioural	22.4
USA	Fox & Stallworth* (2010)	779	Behavioural	64
Norway	Mattheisen et al.,(1989) #	84	Self-Label With Defn	10.3
Norway	Einarsen & Skogstad (1996)	554	Self-Label With Defn	1.9
UK	Hoel & Cooper (2000)	356	Self-Label With Defn	15.6
Lithuania	Malinauskiene et al.,(2005)#	475	Self-Label With Defn	2.6
Sweden	Hansen et al.,(2006)	172	Self-Label With Defn	7
Ireland	O'Connell et al.,(2007)	1260	Self-Label With Defn	25
New Zealand	Bentley et al.,(2009)	459	Self-Label With Defn	5.2
UK	NASUWT* (1995)	na	Self-Labelling	45
UK	Teacher Support Network (2008)	892	Self-Labelling	23.8
UK	Adamson et al.,* (2011)	3,400	Self-Labelling	32
UK	ATL* (2011)	902	Self-Labelling	12
UK	NASUWT* (2011)	3000	Self-Labelling	44
UK	NASUWT * (2012)	3557	Self-Labelling	54.2

* Sample consists of union members.
# Cited by Zapf et al., 2011.

We have taken the average values for the examples given for teachers and compared them with those of Neilsen, Matthiesen & Einarsen, (2010). We note that, for each type of measurement, higher values are found for teachers than for other workers. As expected from Neilsen's work self-labelling without definition produces higher results than self-labelling with definition (Table 2).

Table 2: Comparison of the prevalence (%) of workplace bullying for teachers and for other workers

	Averages for teachers from Table 1	Average for other workers from Neilsen, Matthiesen & Einarsen, (2010)
Self-labelling based on a given definition	11.4%	11.3%,
Behavioural measures	30.2%	14.8%
Self-labelling without a given definition	31.4%	18.1%

Among studies that focus on the prevalence of workplace bullying the over-representation of the education sector seems quite common (Zapf et al., 2011; Blase, Blase, & Du, 2008; O'Connell, Calvert & Watson, 2007; Leymann, 1996). If the prevalence of workplace bullying among teachers is greater than that for the general workforce then we must ask why that is so. Much has been written about factors that might affect levels of workplace bullying. They may be divided into two main groups: individual (such as gender, age, ethnicity, disability) and organisational (such as work environment, motivations to bully and leadership styles).

2.2

Person-related and Individual Factors

Gender

Despite the high number of studies investigating the relationship between gender and workplace bullying, the results appear contradictory and ambiguous.

Some recent studies find that women are more at risk of workplace bullying than men, for example: Alterman, Luckhaupt, Dahlhamer, Ward and Calvert, 2013 (USA); Galanaki and Papalexandris, 2013 (Greece); Fevre, Nichols, Prior and Rutherford, 2009 (UK); Lewis and Gunn, 2007 (UK); O'Connell, Calvert and Watson, 2007 (Ireland). However, in 2003 in a Europe wide review of workplace bullying data, although Di Martino, Hoel and Cooper (2003) concluded that, in the majority of cases, women were more likely to be bullied than men, they also suggested that women may be more vulnerable than men simply because of their concentration in high-risk occupations such as nursing, teaching and social work, thus linking gender differences to the type of employment (Di Martino, Hoel & Cooper, 2003).

Other researchers have found no significant gender differences (Trepanier Fernet & Austin, 2013, Canada; Hogh, Hoel & Carneiro, 2011, Denmark; Notelaers, Vermunt, Baillien, Einarsen & De Witte, 2011, Belgium; Bentley et al., 2009, NZ; Hoel & Giga, 2006, UK). Reviewing existing research, Zapf et al., (2011) concluded that there was little evidence that women were at higher risk of bullying than men in relation to gendered attitudes or behaviours, except when they are in a minority in a male dominated organisation; similarly men in a female dominated organisation may be more at risk of bullying.

Johannsdottir and Ofalsson (2004), in Iceland, with a varied sample of 398 workers, found gender differences in strategies for coping with bullying: females sought help and used avoidance strategies more than males, whereas males were more likely to use assertive strategies, and were also more likely to confront the bully. Generally they observed that bullying increased the use of avoidance as a coping strategy and of doing nothing as a response to bullying. Coping strategies appear to be an important factor to consider in an understanding of bullying and will be returned to below.

Studies involving teachers mostly find no significant difference in terms of gender (NASUWT, 2012, UK; McCormack et al., 2009, China; Cemaloglu, 2007, Turkey) although a small number suggest that female teachers are more likely to be bullied than male teachers (Adamson, Owen & Dhillon 2011, UK; Bentley et al., 2009; Blase, Blase & Du, 2008, USA). However none have come to light to suggest that male teachers are more likely to be bullied than female ones.

Age

Fevre, Lewis, Robinson and Jones (2012), reviewing research concerning the general workforce, suggest that the relationship between age and bullying is less than conclusive. Einarsen and Skogstad (1996) in Norway, with a large sample of 7986 workers, found that older workers were at greater risk, as did Hoel and Giga (2006) in a UK survey of 1041 employees, but Notelaers et al., (2011) observed that the youngest employees (those less than 25 yr of age) and the oldest employees (those above 54 yr of age) are least likely to be bullied at work, whereas respondents between 35 and 44 yrs of age had the highest risk. Johannsdottir and Olafsson (2004) in Iceland observed that there was an increased tendency with age to do nothing when faced with bullying.

In research specifically concerning the bullying of teachers we, similarly, find little clear agreement. In Croatia, Russo, Milić, Knežević, Mulić and Mustajbegović (2008) found that younger teachers were more bullied than were older ones. But in Australia, Riley, Duncan and Edwards (2011) found that older teachers (aged over 51) were affected more than younger teachers. Two surveys for NASUWT in the UK also suggest that older teachers are more likely to be at risk: Adamson, Owen and Dhillon, (2011) found that those aged between 40-49 are the most likely to be bullied, and an NASUWT survey (2012) recorded that teachers aged 30 or below are less likely to be the victims of bullying. Bentley et al., (2009) in New Zealand, and Blasé, Blasé and Du, (2008) in the USA suggest that the oldest (aged over 60) and youngest (aged under 30) teachers are most at risk. McCormack, Casimir, Djurkovic and Yang (2009), with a small sample of 142 Chinese teachers, and Cemaloglu, (2007) with a larger sample of 315 Primary school teachers in Turkey, found no significant relationship. Such inconsistency suggests that age alone may not be the main issue, and that perhaps the cultural context and teachers' lived work environments may affect the way teachers of different ages are treated.

In schools in England, older teachers' apparent greater vulnerability may in part relate to regulations on pay and conditions, where older teachers have been inherently more expensive. It has been suggested that some Headteachers may try to reduce their costs by finding ways of getting rid of older teachers and employing younger, cheaper ones in their place (Troman, 2001). As Earnshaw, Ritchie, Marchington, Torrington and Hardy, (2002:33) point out 'staff reductions are a quick way to reduce budget deficits'.

Minority groups

Although workers across Europe are now legally protected from discrimination by law, studies consistently indicate that being part of a minority group, for example, a member of an ethnic minority, a male or female as a minority in the workforce, or having a disability or a chronic illness such as depression increases the risk of workplace bullying.

UK anti-discrimination legislation (Office for Disability Issues, HM Government, 2010), in line with European law, makes it unlawful to discriminate against anyone because of: race, including colour; nationality, ethnic or national origin; religion, belief or lack of religion/belief; sex, sexual orientation or disability (and a number of other groupings) when at work. However, a number of recent UK studies show that respondents from minority ethnic groups are at greater risk of bullying than others (Giga, Hoel & Lewis, 2008a; Lewis & Gunn, 2007; Hoel & Giga, 2006). This effect has also been observed within the teaching profession (Adamson, Owen & Dhillon 2011). However Union officials, during interviews with us, suggested that recent legislation had led to teachers from minority ethnic groups labelling their ill-treatment as racial harassment rather than bullying.

Disability and ill-health

Research from many countries has shown that people who experience bullying are significantly more likely to report negative mental health outcomes, such as anxiety and depression, than those who are not considered bullied, see for example: Trepanier, Fernet and Austin, 2013 (Canada); Neilsen and Einarsen, 2012 (International – meta-analyses of 54 cross – sectional studies and 13 longitudinal studies); Neilsen, Hetland,

Matthiesen and Einarsen, 2012 (Norway); Zapf, Knorz and Kulla, 1996 (Germany). Studies from the UK support this view (TSN, 2008; Hoel & Giga, 2006; Cooper, Hoel & Faragher 2004; Quine, 2001).

However, longitudinal studies suggest an alternative viewpoint: that people with mental and physical health problems may be more likely to report bullying or be more vulnerable to bullying in the first place. Neilsen and Einarsen, (2012), and Neilsen, Hetland, Matthiesen and Einarsen, (2012) showed that having pre-existing mental health problems significantly increased the risk of later bullying, but also that workplace bullying is significantly related to the later development of mental health problems among employees. Recent UK studies corroborate these observations, finding that disabled employees and those with long-term illnesses, especially those with 'psychological' rather than 'physical' illnesses and disabilities, are more likely to experience bullying at work (Carter et al., 2013; Fevre, Lewis, Robinson & Jones, 2011), while Fevre, Robinson, Lewis and Jones (2013) also note that their survey respondents attributed their ill-treatment to the nature of their workplace, rather than to stigma or discrimination.

These findings are supported by the evidence from a number of qualitative studies, including Cunningham, James, and Dibben, (2004) and Foster (2007), who provided important insights into the treatment of employees with disabilities or ill-health, either pre-existing or resulting from bullying. Their work suggests that ill-treatment, including unfair treatment, arises from the way in which organisations manage sickness absence and their responses to anti-discrimination legislation.

Foster's study focused on 20 public sector workers in the UK and included six teachers; other UK research (Rothi, Leavey & Loewenthal, 2010) has focused entirely on the mental health of teachers. Rothi, Leavey and Loewenthal used in-depth interviews with 39 teachers and 6 school leaders to explore the experiences of teachers with work related stress and mental health problems. They found that teachers in the UK believe that their job is highly stressful and results in psychological disorder as well as physical ill-health. They cite a number of factors that impact upon teachers' mental health, including high workload, unsupportive workplaces, bad school management, unacceptable or bullying behaviour from senior leaders and lack of support from management. The authors make a number of recommendations; among these are that the cumulative impact of accountability systems in schools are reviewed, and that high quality support and training for senior leaders, which would include the emotional support of colleagues, needs to be established. The teachers themselves *'recounted incidents of inadequate support, bullying and unacceptable conduct from Senior Managers, Headteachers in particular. Many attributed this behaviour as motivated by a desire for resignation'* (Rothi, Leavey & Loewenthal, 2010:39).Their interviews with school leaders revealed that although they attempted to tailor their responses to the needs of each individual teacher, putting extra support in place where possible, they were concerned about what could feasibly be done given the financial costs of long term classroom support. Some felt that the current system leads to a deterioration of staff support: *'The school system and its activities lack transparency and this has a tendency to permit bad management practice.'* (Op. Cit. p.39)

Rothi, Leavey and Loewenthal's 2010 research supports that of Cunningham, James and Dibben (2004) and Foster (2007) in demonstrating the difficulty of supporting teachers suffering from ill-health in schools, which is often at odds with the injunction of support, due mainly to lack of resources and lack of training.

Ill-health among UK teachers has also been shown to accompany Capability issues to a large extent. For example, Earnshaw et al., (2002) found that: *'One out of every two teachers confronted with issues related to their Capability were subsequently absent through sickness and in the vast majority of cases the absence was due to a stress-related illness.'* (Earnshaw et al., 2002:42).

The use of Capability Procedures (CPs) is discussed below, in Section 2.3

Occupational status and power

Power disparity between perpetrator and target is usually *'central to any definition of bullying'* (Einarsen, Hoel, Zapf & Cooper, 2003: 21).

In many European countries, in the USA and in Australia, studies of workplace bullying show that higher status employees are more likely to be perpetrators of bullying. Research from the UK and Ireland has found that employees are mostly bullied by their superiors (Carter et al., 2013; Fevre, Robinson, Lewis & Jones, 2013; Hoel & Giga, 2006; Quine 2001; O'Moore, Seigne, McGuire & Smith, 1998; Rayner & Hoel, 1997). Among the most recent UK studies, Fevre, Robinson, Lewis and Jones, (2013) observed that employers, line managers or supervisors were said to be responsible for 44.8% of bullying behaviour, and Carter et al.,(2013) working with 2950 UK National Health Service staff found that managers were the most common source of bullying.

Recent USA research by Fox and Stallworth (2010) found that 45.6% of the teachers in their study reported being targets of pervasive bullying by their administrators/principals. Djurovic, McCormack and Casimir (2008) in Australia observed that in the majority of cases, teacher bullying was vertical and downward, with 58% reporting the main perpetrator to be of higher rank while 26% reported that the perpetrator was of the same rank, and 13% that the perpetrator was of lower rank.

A survey by the NASUWT (2011) revealed that 80% of those who bullied occupied leadership or line management posts but an increase in distributed management has resulted in a larger number of Deputies and Heads of department being identified as bullies. However, Adamson, Owen and Dhillon (2011) surveying NASUWT members' experiences, found that although around 56% of their cases of bullying/harassment were perpetrated by the person's immediate line-manager just over a third were perpetrated by a colleague (36%). Hoel and Cooper (2000:10) concluded that '*bullying varies greatly between sectors and occupations with employees within the prison service, post and telecommunications, school-teaching and the dance profession being most at risk*'. In further analysis of this data Hoel, Cooper and Faragher (2001: 462) highlighted that bullying '*affects people of all organisational status groups*'.

Later large scale studies of various sectors within the UK agree that '*the main culprit occupies a managerial or supervisory role*' and that this was '*a critical feature of the British pattern of bullying. Most studies report this pattern in 70 to 80 percent of cases*'. (Beale & Hoel, 2010:103)

However, some Scandinavian studies have seen a different picture: Einarsen and Skogstad (1996) report that Norwegian employees were equally bullied by colleagues and superiors. Upwards bullying has also been observed, in which managers are bullied by those reporting to them (Branch, Ramsay & Barker, 2007). This suggests that although formal organisational status in terms of position/hierarchy is important, particularly in the UK and USA, it is not a prerequisite for bullying, and that some bullies may acquire or gain for themselves some informal power over their targets and be prepared to use it improperly.

Coping and resistance

Johannsdottir and Ofalsson (2004) found gender differences in strategies for coping with bullying: males sought help less and used avoidance strategies less than females (and were more likely to use assertive strategies and to confront the bully). They also observed that the use of avoidance as a coping strategy increased with age. The different kinds of coping strategies used by men and women and by different age groups may possibly explain why there is a lack of consistency within the data from different research studies related to gender and age, as well as personality.

Coping with being bullied in the workplace has been the subject of some interesting qualitative research. Lutgen-Sandvik (2006) wrote about coping in terms of 'resistance strategies'. These included:

- Leaving, intentions/threats to leave, transfers/requests for transfers.
- Mutual Advocacy – developing shared action plans, backing up peers and protecting co-workers/subordinates.
- Grievance procedures.
- Documentation – keeping written records of abusive interactions.
- Resistance-through-distance, which dissociates or removes workers both physically and communicatively from bullies.
- Retaliation, where participants verbalize desires for vengeance or reciprocation of injury in kind.
- Confrontation, face-to-face with the bully or public challenges through humorous retorts.
- Research Interview – where participation in the research project was a type of resistance.

Lutgen-Sandvik's data came not from teachers but from a group of 30 other employees within the USA. However a few qualitative works do focus specifically on teachers and include reference to the coping strategies teachers use (Fahie & Devine, 2012; De Wet, 2010; Lewis, 2004).

The most detailed account of coping strategies among teachers comes from Fahie and Devine (2012) who obtained data from in-depth interviews with 24 teachers in Ireland. They include: leaving the school, contacting their union confidentially, seeking support from family and colleagues, or more overt action such as taking legal action.

Research by Lewis (2004) in the UK had a different focus, investigating how bullying at work led to feelings of guilt and shame among 15 university and college lecturers and Further Education teachers. However, some of his respondents did refer to actions which were in fact coping strategies: speaking of leaving and about approaching their union, adding that they were unwilling to use the available procedures despite union support, mainly due to the fear of future intimidation.

Personality

A wide range of personality traits among victims of bullying have been suggested. Victims have been variously described as: conscientious, over-achieving, introverted, and unrealistic (Einarsen, 1999), and as having lower levels of self-esteem and social capability than non-targets (Einarsen, 2000). In contrast, other studies have indicated that many victims of bullying have no distinctive personality characteristics (Glasø, Matthiesen, Nielsen & Einarsen, 2007; Djurkovic, McCormack & Casimir, 2006; Matthiesen & Einarsen, 2001; Zapf, 1999), while Leymann and Gustafsson (1996) suggest that personality differences between targets and non-targets of bullying may be a consequence and not a cause of bullying.

Glasø, Matthiesen, Nielsen and Einarsen, (2007: 318), working with two matched groups of bullied and non-bullied respondents in Norway, found that, for the most part, the bullied and non-bullied were quite alike as far as personality was concerned. However they concluded that:

> 'Personality should not be neglected being an important factor in understanding the bullying phenomenon. Yet, personality does not easily differentiate targets from non-targets. Hence, the main focus when intervening in order to prevent bullying in organisations must be on organisational factors more than on the personality of victims.'

Thus the issue of personality in relation to bullying remains unresolved.

The literature and research evidence suggests that an individual's age, gender and personality characteristics should not be regarded as major factors affecting workplace bullying, but that being a member of a minority group, having a disability or ill-health do appear to be important. In general, no clear profile of either bullies or targets has emerged (Di Martino, Hoel & Cooper, 2003) although in the UK the perpetrators are more likely to hold a higher position within the organisation. What is clear is that there are consistent differences in the prevalence of bullying in different organisations/workplaces. Thus it seems likely that workplace environment itself is a major factor.

2.3

Work Environment and Organisational Factors

Leymann's work environment hypothesis, in 1992, proposed that bullying was primarily a consequence of prevailing environmental conditions within organisations, rather than particular characteristics of the targets (Hauge, Skogstad & Einarsen, 2007; Einarsen, Raknes & Matthiesen, 1994), and suggests that the bullying process is fuelled by stressful and discordant work environments that might include, for example, inadequate work organisation, ineffective leadership practices and/or stressful jobs (Leymann, 1996).

Levels of bullying vary considerably between organisational sectors (O'Connell, Calvert & Watson, 2007; Lehto & Pärnänen, 2007; Hubert & Veldhoven, 2001; Einarsen & Skogstad, 1996). Certain types of organisation are identified as risk areas for workplace bullying, and in most countries the public sector appears more at risk than the private sector (Hoel, 2013; Zapf et al., 2011; Hoel & Giga, 2006; Cooper, Hoel & Faragher, 2004; Hoel & Cooper, 2000; Lee, 2000; Einarsen & Skogstad, 1996) This is particularly so in the UK (Hoel, 2013), with 64% of UK public sector workers likely to report stress (which is related to bullying) as a major concern at work compared to 48% in the private sector (Blaug, Kenyon & Lekhi, 2007). Teaching has been identified as one of the sectors with the highest risks of bullying in the UK (Hoel & Cooper, 2000), and in New Zealand a large-scale survey across health, education and hospitality found that the highest rates of bullying and stress were reported in the education sector (Bentley et al., 2009).

Bullying has been defined as a severe social stressor at work (Zapf, 1999), and workplace bullying has often been attributed to work-related stress (Notelaers, Baillien, De Witte, Einarsen & Vermunt, 2013; O'Connell, Calvert & Watson, 2007). The UK's Health and Safety Executive (HSE, 2014) have defined work related stress as: 'The adverse reaction people have to excessive pressures or other types of demand placed on them at work.' A recent study (Nubling, Vomstein, Nubling & Adiwidjaja, 2011) has shown rather strong differences between levels of stress inside the EU/EFTA countries, and that by far the highest values are obtained in the UK.

Although stress in itself is not an illness, it may lead to the development of mental and physical illness if it becomes excessive and prolonged. There is a rich literature on stress, and the most influential models seem to have evolved from Karasek's 1979 Job Demand-Control model (JDC) in which two aspects of the work environment – job demand and job control – determine the effects of work on the health and stress of the employee. The initial model suggested that strain on employees was greatest where demands of the job were high and employees had little control over what they did. A later modification, the Job Demand-Control-Support model (JDCS), included the role played by social support at work (Karasek & Theorell, 1990). Research by the Health and Safety Executive (HSE) led to the development of a set of management standards based on the JDCS model. These standards identify six key sources of stress: Demands, Control, Support, Relationships, Organisational Change and Role Stressors (Cousins, MacKay, Kelly, Lee & McCaig, 2004). More recently Notelaers et al., (2013) have linked workplace bullying to particular aspects of the JDCS model with results showing that the likelihood of being a target of severe bullying was more strongly related to job control than to job demands.

In the education sector in New Zealand risk factors identified by Bentley et al., (2009) include organisational or situational factors, with dysfunctional leadership and poor management perceived as the main risk factors by all the respondents. Workplace stress research in the UK (Blaug, Kenyon & Lekhi, 2007) has found that workload is the most pervasive factor linked to work-related stress. Factors other than workloads alone include cuts in staff, change, long hours, bullying, shift work and sexual or racial harassment. But where managers are seen as supportive, employees are significantly less likely to be absent or report stress–induced illness behaviour (Seymour & Grove, 2005).

Schools are small parts of much larger educational systems. Governments in different countries produce legislation which has both direct and indirect effects on their schools, and the leaders and workforces in them. At the macro level in the UK the Department for Education (DFE)[5] is an arm of government. Beneath the DFE, at the meso-level, are LAs and other organisations such as businesses and churches that have oversight of large numbers of schools. At the micro-level are the individual schools themselves. School leaders and teachers work within these micro environments which are largely structured and shaped at the macro level by the prevailing government. There are two major driving forces at work affecting the school environment: firstly, the constraining structures imposed externally, within which teachers and their leaders must work, such as the post-ERA context outlined above, and secondly, the agencies and freedoms that teachers and school leaders have within their individual school settings.

The traditional hierarchical structure of schools lies always within that broader context and leads to power differentials.

---

5   Apart from specific references the initials DFE are used throughout for simplicity, although the name and initials change regularly with changing governments

Of the six HSE stressors (Cousins et al., 2004), the first four (change, demand, control and role stressors) are strongly mediated by both external structures and the leadership or management in individual schools, with the best school leaders able in some ways to mitigate external effects on staff. The last two HSE stressors, support and relationships, fall primarily within the remit of school leaders and managers, allowing direct impact on the stress levels of staff. School leaders and managers do have some control over how national changes are implemented in their schools but they are also affected by external controls on them, such as the threat to Headteachers' jobs if performativity and quality standards fail to meet Ofsted criteria, or the need to manage staff in the light of reduced budgets or falling rolls.

HSE key stressors are insufficient in themselves for a full understanding of the workplace bullying of teachers. However, there is considerable evidence that these factors do impact on teachers' working lives, in particular on their levels of work stress, but also on their experiences of bullying. In the next section, research concerning teachers' stress and bullying is considered, first in terms of 3 of the JDCS factors (Demand, Control and Support) as starting points, followed by an examination of Relationships, Role and Change in schools.

Demand, Control and Support

Survey data across schools in 27 European countries, including the UK (Billehøj, 2007) suggest that demands on teachers have grown in terms of increased workload, role overload, increased class sizes and increasing incidents of unacceptable pupil behaviour. The prevailing workplace environment within schools in the UK has changed radically post-ERA, with much increased levels of workload (DFE, 2014), accountability, micro-management, overt supervision and work intensity. Despite a series of 'remodelling' initiatives designed to liberate teachers from onerous workloads (Galton & MacBeath, 2008), workload remains a major concern for teachers in England. According to NASUWT (2014) workload has risen from 74% in 2011 to 78% in 2013, while increased workload is making the greatest contribution to levels of teacher stress in Scotland (Mulholland, McKinlay & Sproule 2013).

As explained above, external quality assurance and performance monitoring of schools in England is extensive and pervasive, while the National Curriculum prescribes what is to be taught in state schools that remain under LA control. Teaching as a profession, in this 21st Century, is characterised as being highly subject to external control and regulation (Hargreaves et al., 2007). Centrally driven education policies are also subject to frequent change, depending upon which political party is in power:

> 'A paradox of the current position is that despite the persistent and growing emphasis on autonomy most school practitioners consider themselves significantly constrained by government requirements to an extent that is undoubtedly far greater than their forbears in 1975 would have done. The last quarter century in particular has been a time of continuous policy change' (Glatter, 2012: 564).

The performative culture that surrounds UK schools, and the power differences implicit within their increasingly hierarchical management systems, brings issues of control and autonomy to the fore. There is some limited evidence that UK teachers feel they have lower levels of control than other professions (Grenville-Cleave & Boniwell, 2012), and a small study by Griva and Joekes (2003) observed that UK teachers had lower control than teachers in other European countries. In a large UK study,

Hargreaves et al.,(2007: 9) stated that: *'In general, the teaching profession sees itself as lacking in reward and respect but highly characterised by external control and regulation compared with a high status profession.* A survey of the effects of policy changes on English Primary teachers' practice by Galton and MacBeath (2002: 64) reported that *'Increasing prescription from above was seen* [by teachers] *as bringing with it a loss of control, initiative and imagination'.*

The current accountability systems in education put pressure on, and make it more acceptable for, school leaders and their managers to use their positional power to control teachers and shape their work. Leaders' control includes CPs, which the NASUWT (2011: 6) observed, *'appear to be used as a tool to bully some teachers, particularly those in the latter stages of their teaching careers'.*

Heads and Senior Managers are subject to similar external constraints, prescriptions and judgements as are their staff (and more besides). In addition there are rules which affect the amount of financial support provided to individual schools, alongside employment and sickness rights. The inflexibility and uncertainty over funding means there is a likelihood of increased use of non-teaching staff instead of qualified teachers, as described by Sibieta (2015). Higham and Earley's (2013) survey of school leaders from 1006 schools in England found that the two most significant leadership challenges anticipated over the next 18 months were reductions in funding and a new Ofsted inspection framework.

Day and Sammons (2013: 8) noted that: *'Headteachers' professional associations have called for more intelligent accountability, more flexibility on staff pay and conditions'* and, in particular, *'more support and less pressure'* for school leaders from national agencies, Ofsted and central government.

Leader or manager support within schools has been shown to be an important factor mitigating the effects of stress and bullying, and reducing the likelihood of teachers leaving/ resigning (Hogh, Hoel & Carneiro, 2011; McCormack, Casimir, Djurkovic & Yang, 2009; Djurkovic, McCormack & Casimir, 2008). The same authors have indicated the importance of supportive leadership and have confirmed that it is likely to be central to the improvement of teacher wellbeing. Van Dick and Wagner (2001: 256) found that the negative impact of stress on teachers could be buffered through such support and noted that: '...the positive influence of principal support has political impact: if the school principal has a key function in mediating between teachers' needs and demands of the educational system which often are unavoidably stressful, he or she should be well prepared to fit this role.' Studies in Canada (Butt & Retallick, 2002) and Belgium (Aelterman, Engels, Petegem & van Verhaeghe, 2007) found that when teachers felt their leaders provided encouragement and support those leaders were also able to create a more positive organisational climate, which moderated workplace bullying and intention to leave teaching.

A report for the GTCE argues strongly that lack of supportive leadership and inconsistent management practices are at the root of problems surrounding the nature and extent of Capability issues in schools, and that this makes it difficult to reach hard and fast conclusions about the problem (Morrell, Tennant, Kotecha, Newmark & O'Connor, 2010). Research also shows that the vast majority of teachers who are subject to CPs resign without them being completed (Earnshaw et al., 2002). Union representatives have voiced concerns about how Heads operate the CPs, which are intended to be supportive of improvement in a teacher's practice. They question how genuinely supportive the procedure is, with CPs often being used as a tool to remove a teacher from the school. They believed that some Heads did not follow the procedures and that support for the teacher was not always as comprehensive as it should be. Some also felt that CPs were being used where a teacher had been in conflict with the Head rather than via evidence of poor professional practice (Earnshaw et al., 2002).

In a review of the evidence concerning Capability the NASUWT concluded that CPs were disproportionately applied in relation to older teachers, male teachers and disabled teachers. They also suggested that the way school managers understand and interpret Capability may be strongly affected by factors outside individual teachers' control and that CPs are *'initiated disproportionately with teachers aged over 50 years'* (NASUWT, 2011:10), while Earnshaw et al.,(2002:11) suggested that Heads and Union officials felt that *'the use of Capability procedures was inappropriate in the case of teachers in their '50s who had performed satisfactorily in the past'*. Those aged 51 to 60 are usually more expensive to employ than younger and less experienced teachers, and they experience a far greater degree of adult workplace bullying (DFE, 2013; Adamson, Owen & Dhillon, 2011; Troman & Woods, 2001). A NASUWT survey (2012) revealed that 80% of those who bully occupy leadership or line management posts, confirming research by the Education Support Partnership (TSN, 2008), which also found that Headteachers and Senior Managers were the main perpetrators of bullying. Their ability to threaten, or to actually put teachers into Capability may go some way to explain this.

Demand, Control and Support, as workplace environment stressors of teachers, may help to explain the higher risk of bullying experienced by teachers. However a model proposed by Salin (2003) allows bullying to be understood somewhat differently, in terms of structures and processes that may act as enablers, triggers or motivations for bullying.

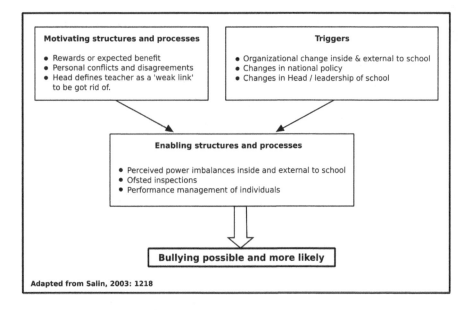

Figure 1: Structures and processes increasing likelihood of bullying (Adapted from Salin, 2003:1218)

As Figure 1 illustrates, there are:

- **enabling structures,** such as perceived power imbalances inside and external to schools which affect all staff, including Heads, leadership teams and teachers, from Ofsted inspections to performance management of individuals;
- **'triggers' or precipitating processes,** such as organisational change inside and external to schools, which affect all staff, from changes in national policy to changes in Headteacher/ leadership of school; and
- **motivating structures,** such as expected benefits or rewards, personal conflicts and disagreements, or a teacher defined by the Headteacher as a 'weak link' to be got rid of.

Salin concluded that bullying is often the result of an interaction between structures and processes from all three groupings. As we shall see below her model is very helpful in understanding how some organisational conditions might lead to bullying within the education sector and how the remaining HSE stressors (relationships, role stressors and change) might be involved in this.

Power and relationships, role stressors and change

The power imbalance between organisations and their individual employees is an enabling structure for bullying, with organisations themselves sometimes being perceived by their employees as bullies (Liefooghe & Mackenzie Davey, 2001). However, since power is also defined as an action, something enacted rather than merely held, the possibility of power being negatively exercised often (but not always) lies in a disparity in the ability to exercise power. Thus immediate supervisors and managers are often the most likely to be perceived or experienced as bullies given the direction of hierarchical power differentials.

All Headteachers, including those who bully, are, in some ways, constrained by and subject to external conditions over which they may have little or no control: they are publicly accountable for the effective use of public funds and the overall quality of their school, and they are accountable to parents and the pupils themselves. However they also have hierarchical power in their schools, a positional power which is shared with their governing bodies (Bubb, Earley & Totterdell 2005) at the micro-level of the school.

A survey of Australian teachers, most of whom had experienced workplace bullying, found that a power imbalance due to job position was a major factor in workplace bullying behaviour (Riley, Duncan, & Edwards, 2009), while in South Africa De Wet (2010) noted that bullying thrives in organisations that are hierarchic, bureaucratic and/or rule-orientated. In an international review of the literature on school improvement Lindahl (2007:325) identifies an issue with the

distribution of power regarding national school improvement
policies and the role of school leaders:

> *'...if power over decision-making related to school
> improvement is held primarily at the national, state or
> local education agency level, and not shared with the
> school, any proposed changes will be viewed as externally
> imposed, invoking resistance in even otherwise healthy
> school cultures. In such cases leaders are faced with the
> choice of supporting the externally proposed changes and
> facilitating the school's acceptance of them or of resisting
> them, with the attendant consequences.'*

Role stressors, the last of Cousins et al's., (2004) 6 key stressors,
represent expectations and demands from those in more
hierarchically powerful positions. They include **role ambiguity**,
where there is insufficient or uncertain information from
superiors about what is expected, and **role conflict**, which
involves the simultaneous existence of two or more sets of
expectations, so that fulfilling one makes fulfilment of the other
difficult. These types of role stressors in work environments are
enabling processes (Fig. 1) that can lead to bullying situations
(Baillien, Neyens, De Witte & De Cuyper, 2009; Roscigno, Lopez
& Hodson, 2009; Hauge, Skogstad & Einarsen, 2007).

In the public service sector Strandmark and Hallberg (2007)
observe that conflicting values in the workplace may occur
due to poor organisational conditions, and weak or indistinct
leadership, while De Wet (2014:14) argues that: *'Bullying is
likely to occur in schools where organisational chaos reigns. Such
schools are characterised by incompetent, unprincipled, abusive
leadership, lack of accountability, fairness and transparency.'*

Lack of clarity around work roles and goals, and inadequate
information and communication are linked to bullying (Baillien
& De Witte, 2009; Matthiesen & Einarsen, 2007; Strandmark

& Hallberg, 2007; Agervold & Mikkelsen, 2004; Einarsen, 1999; Vartia, 1996) while poor communication, deliberate miscommunication (which is a bullying strategy), or conflicts that affect information flow are all also associated with bullying (Zapf, 1999), and such conditions are likely to be present in chaotic or poorly managed organisations.

When compared with other leaders or managers Headteachers are found to suffer significantly higher levels of stress and stress-related illness (Howard, 2012; Phillips, Sen & McNamee, 2008). Philips, Sen & McNamee (2007) found that 43% of their sample of Headteachers reported work related stress, and the National Association of Head Teachers (NAHT) Work-Life Balance Survey in 2008/2009 (French, 2009), recorded 85% of their sample as experiencing work related stress. The latter report went on to state that 64% of respondents believed that they had suffered illness as a result. Howard's results (2012) in a Doctoral thesis supported these findings. The top sources of stress for Headteachers found by Howard (2012), French (2009) and Philips, Sen and McNamee (2007) were workload and Ofsted/HMI inspection.

Headteachers have to deal with high levels of accountability in schools (MacBeath, 2011; Bristow, Ireson & Coleman, 2007), high demands (Bristow, Ireson & Coleman, 2007; Price Waterhouse Coopers, 2007), isolation (MacBeath, 2011; Bristow, Ireson & Coleman, 2007; Bright & Ware, 2003) and, over the last few years, fear of losing their job if their school does not meet ever more stringent conditions (MacBeath, 2011; Earley, Weindling, Bubb & Glenn, 2009). Many school leaders feel the need for better support (Woods, Woods & Cowie, 2009; Bristow, Ireson & Coleman, 2007; Bright & Ware, 2003), and evidence suggests they are struggling to meet all the demands currently placed on them (Price Waterhouse Coopers, 2007).

Professional development that focused on dealing with underachieving staff and managing and evaluating learning and teaching would be welcomed by Scottish Heads (Woods, Woods & Cowie, 2009) as it would enhance their ability to lead and manage their schools and staff effectively and fairly, and it could help them develop survival strategies for the many stresses of their role, including the conflicting demands made on them.

> *"Coping' is a word that carries a sense of struggle, swimming with the current, keeping one's head above water. These were the kind of metaphors used by Scottish Heads to depict their situation. Pressure and constant demands 'from above' (in itself a telling metaphor for the hierarchical nature of the relationship between schools, local authorities and government) was a common theme.'*
> MacBeath, O'Brien & Gronn (2012: 428)

Only a few of MacBeath, O'Brien and Gronn's Headteachers had been provided with support, mentoring or leadership programmes. Robbins (2013) aimed to find evidence of training in the UK to provide school leaders with the strategies necessary to cope with work related stress. However, his survey of all the main training institutions in the UK, between September 2010 and July 2011, found a distinct lack of any courses that specifically prepared school leaders for the stress of their roles.

Organisational change

At the meso and micro levels many studies demonstrate that organisational change can create workplace climates where bullying by managers is more likely (e.g. Beale & Hoel, 2011; Hauge et al., 2011; Skogstad, Matthiesen & Einarsen, 2007). The majority of the very many macro-level changes in English education have been brought about by political actions external to schools (Evans, 2011; Wilkins, 2011) and subsequent to the1988 ERA (Webb, Vulliamy, Hämäläinen & Poikonen, 2012; MacBeath & Galton, 2008; Brown & Ralph, 2002). The effects of these changes, at least on Primary teachers were profound, with teachers describing '*the undermining effects of imposed change and, in its wake, the devaluing of the teacher's professional worth*' (Galton & MacBeath, 2002: 63).

Organisational changes, be they in management or the work group, are triggers for bullying (Hoel & Cooper, 2000; O'Moore, Seigne, McGuire & Smith, 1998; Rayner & Hoel, 1997): in a study by O'Moore, Seigne, McGuire & Smith (1998) almost two-thirds of the victims stated that the bullying commenced after the promotion of the perpetrator or the arrival of a new manager. The transition from one Headteacher to another is a major change in school organisation: Bird (2008), writing from the perspective of English Secondary schools suggests that the presence of a new Headteacher can lead to a troubled staff and, according to Illingworth (2010), an increased risk of bullying. McMahon's (2001) case study of an English Primary school found that change of leadership could have a substantial negative effect: after the departure of one Headteacher, four successor Headteachers, acting or substantive over a period of 4 years led, according to Ofsted, to '*a period of instability caused by difficulties in the leadership and management*' (p.102), and this was reflected in a drop in SATs scores, pupil behaviour problems, poor staff communication and '*a breakdown in relationships between the Headteacher and the senior management team*' (p.109).

Motivations for bullying

Alongside triggers and enablers, Salin (2003:1222) suggests that '*there are certain motivating circumstances that can actually make it rewarding to harass others in the workplace*'. It is argued (Beale & Hoel, 2011) that leaders may benefit significantly from bullying, for example where high performance work practices are demanded. Bullying by managers may be conscious and rational: for example Ferris et al., (2007:197) proposed that bullying may be a strategic attempt to increase the bully's power and reputation, and to increase the job performance not only of the targets, but also of those around them. They suggested that *'leader bullying represents strategically selected tactics of influence by leaders designed to convey a particular image and place targets in a submissive, powerless position whereby they are more easily influenced and controlled, in order to achieve personal and/or organisational objectives.'*

It has also been argued that managers and supervisors may use a form of bullying to achieve organisational goals, and thereby improve and protect their own status and prospects of advancement. In their review of the individual antecedents of bullying Zapf and Einarsen, (2011:185) conclude that managers do indeed profit *'by using bullying as a form of micro-political behaviour'*. Salin and Hoel (2011) argue that in some very competitive work environments bullying may also be used strategically to get rid of over or under-achieving colleagues or subordinates who are considered either threats or burdens. These authors (p.234) cite work by Zapf and Warth which indicates that bullying may be *'personnel work by other means'*, and may be used to get rid of certain unwanted employees whom it would otherwise be difficult to remove. It has also been suggested that higher rates of bullying within the public sector may result from the rules and legal requirements that make it more difficult to get rid of certain employees (Salin, 2001; O'Moore, 2000).This idea is supported by Lee (2000), who has observed that bullying may be used as a way of getting rid of staff without making redundancy payments. External financial controls, which in English state schools are dependent on the number of pupils on roll and Government budgets, can provide the occasion, a medium and a rationale for managerial bullying

(Armstrong 2011). With older teachers more expensive to employ than younger and less experienced ones (DFE, 2013; Adamson, Owen & Dhillon, 2011; Troman, 2001), age might be a factor.

2.4

Leadership Style

Research evidence indicates that organisational leadership is an especially critical risk factor for the occurrence of workplace bullying (Hoel, Glasø, Hetland, Cooper & Einarsen, 2010; Hershcovis, Turner, Barling, Arnold, Dupré, Inness, LeBlanc & Sivanathan, 2007). Leadership definitions and descriptions vary enormously, and include management models, philosophies and styles (Bush & Glover, 2003). There is no single agreed or correct definition of the concept of leadership, '*Like all constructs in social sciences, the definition of leadership is arbitrary and very subjective. Some definitions are more useful than others*' (Yukl, 1994, cited by Leithwood, Jantzi & Steinbach, 1999:5).

Leadership styles, which classify or describe the ways in which leaders behave, have been the subject of extensive research that has been linked both positively and negatively to the risk of workplace bullying. In the 1940s Kurt Lewin's seminal leadership theory proposed three styles of leadership: authoritarian, participative and laissez-faire. Using an authoritarian (or autocratic) leadership style the leader spells out the goals, deadlines and methods, making decisions alone, with little or no consultation. Leaders who adopt this style can go too far and can be seen by others as over-controlling and dictatorial. Leaders using a participative (or democratic) style express their priorities and values in setting goals and making decisions, but also accept advice and suggestions from colleagues, although the leader makes the final decision. Laissez-faire leadership refers to the avoidance or absence of leadership and is considered to be the most inactive as well as the most ineffective leadership style (Bass & Riggio, 2006).

The study of leadership has continued over many decades and a wide range of theories have been developed. One of the best known is the Full Range Model of Leadership (Bass & Riggio, 2006; Avolio, Bass & Jung, 1999), in which leadership style is described on a continuum from passive and ineffective (laissez-faire), through transactional, to active and effective leadership styles such as transformational leadership. Transformational leadership is associated with achieving change through shared goals, and the communication of high expectations which focus followers' attention on long-term vision, facilitate change, and support new ways of working.

Transactional leadership, has been described as a carrot or a stick approach (Bass, 1997), involving motivation by praise and rewards for performance (contingent reward) or correction by negative feedback, reproof, threats, or disciplinary actions (management by exception). Contingent reward leaders engage in a constructive transaction of reward for performance, clarifying expectations, and providing approval of successful performance. Management by exception leaders monitor performance and take corrective action if deviations from standards occur: they enforce rules to avoid mistakes. Bass (1997) describes a hierarchy among these leadership styles in terms of their effectiveness, effort, and satisfaction (see Fig. 2 below). Transformational leaders are the most effective; contingent reward is somewhat more effective than active management by exception, which in turn is more effective than passive management by exception, with laissez-faire leadership being the least effective.

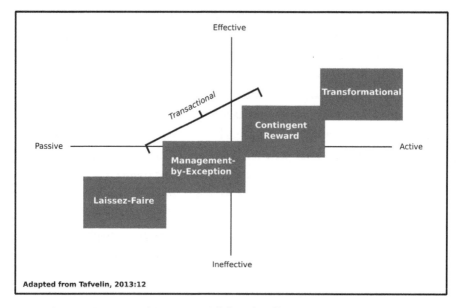

Adapted from Tafvelin, 2013:12

Figure 2: A version of Bass & Riggio's (2006) Full Range Leadership Model adapted from Tafvelin, 2013:12

According to Bass (1997) transformational leaders can display both transformational and transactional behaviour; they can be directive or participative, authoritarian or democratic because context and culture affect their behaviour.

Reviews of the literature have concluded that certain leadership styles lead to a greater risk of bullying (Illing et al., 2013; Krasikova, Green & LeBreton, 2013), with workplace bullying tending to occur in organisations characterized by autocratic management styles (Erturten, Cemalcilar & Aycan, 2012; Agervold, 2009; Hoel & Cooper, 2000; O'Moore, 2000; Vartia, 1996). Autocratic leadership is often used synonymously with directive or coercive styles, and concepts such as 'abusive supervision' (Harris, Harvey, Harris & Cast, 2013; Tepper, 2000) or 'tyrannical leadership' (Einarsen, Aasland & Skogstad, 2007) have been used to describe this style. Destructive leadership is associated not only with lack of effectiveness in carrying out the leader role, but also with damaging experiences for subordinates (Schyns & Schilling, 2013; Hoel et al., 2010). Similarly, laissez faire leadership styles can also contribute to a climate of workplace bullying; empirical findings associate it with interpersonal conflicts and bullying (Neilsen, 2013; Hoel et al., 2010; Hauge, Skogstad & Einarsen, 2007; Skogstad, Einarsen, Torsheim, Aasland & Hetland, 2007; Nielsen, Matthiesen & Einarsen, 2005). However, transformational leadership has been linked to more positive work environments and reduced risk of bullying (Tafvelin, 2013; Erturten, Cemalcilar & Aycan, 2012; Gholamzadeh & Khazaneh, 2012). Thus the evidence available strongly supports the idea that certain leadership styles directly affect the risk of workplace bullying, although there are few studies that relate directly to schools.

Of these, bullying has been linked to an authoritarian leadership style in Primary schools in two small South African studies by De Wet (2010, 2014), and to laissez-faire leadership in Secondary and tertiary educational establishments in a large New Zealand survey by Bentley et al., (2009). An authoritarian style, often referred to as paternalistic (where the leader shows both autocratic and nurturing behaviours), was also found to be a significant predictor of workplace bullying for teachers in Primary schools in Turkey (Cerit, 2013).

Two further studies from Turkey investigated the relationship between organisational health and leadership styles, this time focusing on transformational and transactional styles (Cemaloglu, 2011; Korkmaz, 2007). Both authors link higher levels of transformational leadership with more positive organisational health for a school, and Cemaloglu (2011) also links it with a reduction in workplace bullying of teachers.

In their review of the school leadership literature Bush and Glover (2003) noted an interest in transformational leadership but found few empirical studies, particularly in the UK context, about the nature of leadership and the relative efficacy of different approaches. Later, Leithwood and Jantzi (2006) used a school-specific model of transformational leadership practices in a study with over 2000 teachers from 655 English Primary schools, demonstrating that transformational leadership had very strong direct effects on teachers' work settings and motivation. But they also pointed out that, '*While there is much discussion in the educational literature, both supportive and critical, about transformational orientations to leadership, empirical evidence about its effects in school contexts is extremely thin*'. (Leithwood & Jantzi, 2006: 204)

Despite the popularity of transformational leadership in the literature the policy climate within UK schools requires school leaders to follow government prescriptions, and '*a more centralised, more directed, and more controlled educational system has dramatically reduced the possibility of realising a genuinely transformational education and leadership*' (Bottery, 2001: 215).

Research by Day, Harris and Hadfield, (2001) suggested that successful Headteachers were both transactional and transformative. More recently Smith and Bell (2011) examined how far Headteachers used transactional or transformational leadership styles and concluded that although Heads use both approaches, and although they believe that transformational leadership is far more effective for successful school development, external pressures cause them to concentrate far more than they would wish on transactional leadership.

2. 5

Conclusion

Constant change post-ERA (DES, 1988) provides the educational context for this research. It includes the imposition of a performative agenda, an increasingly technicist approach to teaching, and a marked reduction in teachers' autonomy and control over their work, all within a system of overt, pervasive and high-stakes accountability.

There have been few qualitative studies into workplace bullying to date, and even fewer that specifically involve teachers, although Salin and Hoel (2011:237) note that *'a few recent studies have applied qualitative research methods, possibly introducing alternative perspectives of the role of organisational antecedents in the bullying process'*. Given the range of definitions and labels applied to workplace bullying, and the lack of clarity about what constitutes workplace bullying, we chose to find out what teachers themselves meant when they said they were being bullied at work, what impact it had on them and what the consequences were for them. This involved a qualitative approach. The nature of our study is outlined in Chapter 3.

3

WHAT WE DID AND WHAT WE FOUND: THE RESEARCH DETAILS

3.1

Our volunteers and our methods

In this chapter we describe the details of our research, and the data from which we fashioned the stories and narratives which form the heart of this book.

We explored the nature and range of teachers' experiences of workplace bullying and what happened as a result, alongside the perspectives of line managers/Heads and professional associations/Unions who deal with it. We wanted to know what was perceived as bullying by the teachers and the impact it had on them. We also wanted to know what school managers and teacher associations thought about it, why they thought it occurred, and what might be done about it. The core data sources are 39 qualitative interviews with teachers who experienced workplace bullying, 10 interviews with Heads/ Deputies, and 7 with teachers' Union officials. All interviews took place in 2012, with volunteers from across England and Wales.

The teachers responded to a request in the weekly e-newsletter of the Education Support Partnership (formerly the TSN) (see appendix). All interested teachers were contacted. They came from all compulsory school phases and levels of seniority, from different schools and geographical areas. Most were from England, though two were from Wales. There were 24 Primary and 15 Secondary teachers aged between 26 and 65; most (27 of 39) were aged 36 to 55, and 35 had at least five years teaching experience (16 had more than 20 years experience). Most had some designated role of responsibility; just 13 had none (for more details see appendix).

The study was explained (including confidentiality of findings/protection of identities), and participants were given an outline of the interview schedule. Most interviews lasted for an hour, primarily one-to-one and face-to-face, although for practical reasons four were conducted by telephone. The teachers chose the location, usually their home, occasionally a coffee shop. The interviews were audio-taped and transcribed verbatim.

We began with demographic questions about age, teaching and other work experiences, and about the school where they felt they had been bullied (see appendix for further details). This was followed by one open question: *Would you please tell me your story?* When the teachers had reached the end of what they wanted to say, three further questions were asked:

- What impact did the bullying have on your professional and/or private life?
- What do you think were the reasons for the bullying?
- What could be done or changed to prevent this from happening to anyone else?

With probes where necessary and follow-up questions, the teachers told their stories, speaking freely, in detail, about their sometimes very upsetting experiences. After the interviews these data were supplemented by related newspaper articles and inspection reports for their schools, which were examined for information about management, school leadership and ethos. Seven teachers also submitted documentation giving additional information. Almost all teachers sent further email updates on their situations the following year and then again two years after their interview. We analysed the data for antecedents, impact and outcomes of bullying for these teachers.

We approached the Unions directly and were offered interviews with 7 senior representatives from four of the major teaching Unions[6]. Initially, we lacked volunteers from senior staff who had to deal with allegations of bullying, but later, through snowball sampling, we acquired and interviewed 10 Heads and Senior Managers (from Primary, Secondary and Middle schools)[7]. These interviews were also face-to-face, lasted about an hour, and were conducted either in their workplace, home or a coffee shop during 2012. We asked for background information about their role and experience in schools, showed them our working definition of bullying (see chapter 1) and then asked them to comment on the extent to which it matched their own experiences, and what, if anything, should be added or omitted from the definition. This led into a general discussion of bullying in schools. We then shared some vignettes with them, based on the experiences of our volunteer teachers, and asked for their comments. In the case of Union officials this also included the range of teacher comments about the response they got from their Union officials when they were being bullied, which led to Union officials talking about the limitations of their power, and about what they saw as the best approaches to take for their members.

Our research is based within a social constructionism perspective, taking *'the view that all knowledge, and therefore all meaningful reality as such, is contingent upon human practices, being constructed in and out of interaction between human beings and their world, and developed and transmitted within an essentially social context'* (Crotty, 1998: 42).

---

6   All the union staff interviewed will be referred to, from this point, as Union Officials

7   All the Headteachers and Deputy Heads interviewed will be referred to, from this point, as 'Senior Managers'

Thus, in our overall approach, we:

- Looked for emerging themes in the interviews to understand the context and the phenomenon of workplace bullying rather than test any predetermined ideas about bullying.
- Gathered participant accounts of workplace bullying in order to understand how it is coped with and understood by those directly affected.
- Identified 'invariant' categories and themes, common elements of experience and differences between sub groups.
- Compared our research findings with theories and constructs presented in the literature.

We took account of the social and educational contexts that significantly shape and frame (but do not determine) our teachers' actions, expectations and experiences and we also looked for any common or shared antecedents, impacts, and outcomes of their bullying experiences, especially in relation to their workplace managers and Union officials.

While we began with teachers' descriptions of their experiences and perceptions, in our later theoretical coding we looked for any links with, and consequences of, particular educational policies, strategies, constraints or opportunities within educational environments.

In focusing on teachers' perceptions, beliefs and understanding, we sought to:

- Identify and describe what teachers regard as workplace bullying.
- Identify who the teachers perceived as bullies.
- Identify the reasons for the bullying as perceived by the teachers.
- Explore new concepts arising from the data.

The data analysis was performed using a Grounded Theory approach, described by Charmaz (2006: 2) as a set of methods that *consist of systematic, yet flexible guidelines for collecting and analyzing qualitative data to construct theories 'grounded' in the data themselves.'*

In a Grounded Theory approach the discovery and labelling of concepts, referred to as 'coding', is the pivotal link between collecting data and developing ideas to explain them. The generation of these ideas is not based on the raw data; it is based on concepts and categories developed out of the raw data. The analysis process involves three stages of data coding:

First, to combine varied raw data, we read the text systematically and meticulously to understand the meaning and the context of the events, identifying themes in the data. The themes were organised under appropriate headings and labels, called codes. We used Nvivo8 computer software to assist in the process.

Then we examined the themes in more detail looking for relationships between categories and subcategories, including conditions, cause-and-effect relationships, and interactions.

For the final stage we integrated categories and subcategories using the central concept of workplace bullying. At this point we decided which themes were most prevalent or important, which contributed most to, and which supported or challenged our analysis. We also looked for exceptions and variations, since purposefully looking for negative cases to refute an idea is as important as looking for supportive data.

These final categories and the relationships between them inform our understanding of the teachers' stories of being bullied and provide valuable insight into the background, circumstances and consequences of their experiences.

3.2

The Teachers' Experiences

All the teachers described to us the bullying they had experienced: most had experienced undermining, verbal abuse, exclusion and/or persistent criticism, and being set unreasonable objectives connected to work overload. Almost half of them felt they had been subject to the unreasonable use of, or threats to use, Capability Procedures (CPs) but few had experienced blocking of professional development and only one had suffered physical abuse.

The following extracts illustrate the types of bullying behaviours most frequently mentioned:

I was giving detentions and stuff like that, the kids would go to her [the Head of Department] *and she would let them off. So anything I was like trying to do was being undermined, and everything I was doing was being criticised… being given a kind of excessive workload. Never being praised for anything… her not communicating what she actually wanted, and then when I did it she would criticise it. She would always find fault.*

(Secondary teacher)

[The Deputy] *just started to rant at me and shout at me, saying – 'this isn't working is it?… And he slated me up and down in front of the TA. He said I wasn't a teacher I was more like a teaching assistant, he couldn't leave me in charge of a class when he was out, and while he was doing this the cleaners appeared in the classroom and he carried on ranting.*

(Primary teacher)

...she was now not speaking to me... basically sent me to Coventry, and anything that she wanted to tell me after school she would send a message through the cleaner.

(Primary teacher)

There were no schemes of work. I was basically writing the schemes of work. I was preparing all the resources. I was getting no help from [the Head of Department] *in terms of that. There was a new syllabus that came in ...GCSE, and I asked for help. But no, I was basically told to do it on my own. It's up to you.*

(Secondary teacher)

A teacher recently graded by Ofsted as 'good with outstanding features' was threatened with a CP:

I was summoned to a completely unexpected meeting with the Head so she could discuss her 'concerns' with me... she believed that my class wouldn't make enough progress over the rest of the year... I was then informed that she intended to take formal proceedings if these things didn't improve... she told me, 'If I take formal proceedings I can no longer give you a good reference... or you can choose to leave while I still can.'

(Primary teacher)

Seventeen teachers were either threatened with, or taken through Competency Procedures. Ten had been threatened with CPs: three resigned, two moving to another teaching post and the other to a non-teaching post; the other seven suffered severe stress-related illness and were on long-term sickness absence. Seven more teachers were taken through the competency process: six of these were on long-term sickness absence suffering from severe stress-related illness. The remaining teacher had been offered a Compromise Agreement to resign but refused it, then resigned and moved to another teaching post.

The seven teachers who actually went through CPs described a procedure that did not comply with that laid down in law. Proper targets had not been set, support was not provided, and in some cases the school had not followed correct procedure in initiating the formal CP:

> ... I had a letter saying they're having a meeting to put me into formal Capability and it was the second to last day of term in July, or I could take this compromise agreement, and take this paltry amount of money and not be back in September, [the Union] advised me not to go to the meeting, because they had not followed procedure... So they put me into formal capabilities in my absence... and about February/March time, I got a letter saying I was no longer in formal Capability, because they hadn't followed procedure.
>
> (Primary teacher)

> I really wanted to be clear so that I would know... And it wasn't [clear]. It was 'Well I'll be able to tell when I walk in the classroom. Well, I'll be able to tell when I walk down the corridor...' It wasn't anything concrete... I kept going back to my Union. The Union thought the action plan was absolutely ludicrous: first of all there were too many targets, second... the ways of meeting the targets did not relate to what the targets were, some of them

were completely beyond my control, some of them were
unachievable in six weeks...

(Primary teacher)

Everything seemed to be going wrong somehow and I
couldn't really work out where I was going wrong, how
things had changed from the previous year to everything
suddenly not being good enough... nothing was put in
writing...There was nothing, everything was verbal...
over that same period there was a member of senior
management who came up to me and said, 'You do know
that there are four of you that she doesn't want in school'.
She came and told me that it had been brought up in a
Senior Management meeting, that there were names of
people who she didn't want in the school... [Later in a
private conversation the Headteacher said to me that]
she was extremely concerned about my Capability and if
I wasn't able to get a job elsewhere and remained within
the school, in September I would be put on informal
Capability procedures... but obviously if I managed to
get myself a job and leave the school before September,
references would be fine and nothing would have to be
said to anybody.

(Primary teacher)

All 17 teachers who commented on how CPs had been threatened, used or abused were working with a new Headteacher.

The Senior Managers and Union officials were divided regarding the use of CPs. Some managers felt that teachers might perceive legitimate situations as bullying whereas Union officials spoke about their potential misuse:

...the thing is that when you get to a certain stage, when
you've done the kind of supportive bit, you actually have

to say these words: 'We're doing this because the ultimate,
you know, the last thing down the line might possibly be,
we would have to look at Capability'. You have to say it
at that point, because you can't leave it unsaid. So, when
you say that, then people see that immediately as a threat.
(Primary Headteacher)

...if a school had concerns... about a teacher, and then
quite rightly wanted to assist in the first place, but felt that
after giving that assistance that there were still issues to be
addressed in a formal sense, from a contractual basis they
should follow [procedure], *but what you find is that...*
they'll either seek to pursue that in a very aggressive way,
undermining the confidence of teachers, or... the teacher
will go sick, long term, and then they'll be managed out of
the system.
(Union official)

Sixteen teachers told us that they were offered a Compromise Agreement (CA), which generally provides a teacher with a fair reference and a sum of money if they resign their post. Nine of these teachers had been threatened with, or taken through CPs, the other 7 were on long-term sick leave as a result of being bullied. Fourteen teachers accepted the CA offered, but two refused the offer and resigned. Four other teachers obtained recompense in terms of payments and apologies or a CA later as a result of legal action.

It was suggested by a number of teachers, Senior Managers and Union officials that some Headteachers used redundancy, CPs and CAs as ways of removing/getting rid of staff. Such routes were likely to be less difficult or costly than having to go through disciplinary or grievance procedures or a tribunal.

I am the principal breadwinner. I contacted the Union,
I've never contacted them before. I was at my wits end.

... I'd had 11 hours of observations that year... At the beginning of the next term – he said he would be coming in to observe me... He was thoroughly unpleasant. He was vindictive. He was just being horrible, he just looked at me with a look of hatred. I felt that his target was to get rid of me.

(Primary teacher)

A new Head came in. It was a little bit prickly generally... there was a bit of an atmosphere in school, she obviously liked some people and she didn't like others, and got rid of two staff fairly quickly... She put a lot of pressure on them, constantly on their backs... They weren't particular friends of mine so I didn't know the details, but I know one of them was got out on Capability and the other one was pushed until he went off with stress. And, this kind of pattern, you kept your head down and you got on with it, and if you did that you were OK, but, looking back, every year one person was pushed out, left through stress or for whatever reason... I feel very strongly that all these new regulations that they are bringing in, about how you can get rid of teachers in a term if they are rubbish, is all well and good getting rid of awful teachers, but it relies on the Head being fair and honest and, in my experience, they are not always. I'm told by my Union that the quality of my teaching was almost irrelevant, the way she handled it, was not done properly. She should not have been behaving like that.

(Primary teacher)

So it was obvious that they wanted me out. Anyway, so, I got onto the Union, told them all about it.

(Secondary teacher)

The school was running a deficit budget and they were looking for staff cuts, either by so-called 'natural wastage' or in any other way... He [the Headteacher] *was looking at senior teachers' salaries, he was looking at getting rid and reducing costs.*

(Primary teacher)

[Finally] *I collapsed and I was terribly, terribly ill. And my husband, Union man and doctors all together said we've got to pull the plug on this. And I ended up signing a compromise agreement, against my better judgement: I hung onto it for ages... the Union would have been happy for me to take the CA, get better and move on.*

(Secondary teacher)

Now I know that, even though you are not supposed to, that you can use redundancy as a means of getting rid of people that you don't want... I've heard lots of Heads say things – Oh I just told him to clear his desk... the maximum you'd get charged at a tribunal, you'd be fined £15,000, which is cheap.

(Secondary Headteacher)

Schools are now, they're getting rid of teachers by using the Capability procedure, because it's easy to do that.

(Union official)

But if they move then into the Capability procedure, it's for us, our people, to ensure that, you know, the alleged underperformance is identified, specifically, so that we know why they're saying that person is under-performing. And then targets set have to be agreed... then it's about identifying the support an employer will give to bring that person up to where they need to be, and an appropriate

*time scale in which to do that. So essentially they're the
elements of the process any employer should follow... if
they go through that and they seem to by and large meet
in full or in part all those various obligations, and at the
end of it an employer still takes the view that that person
is not capable of teaching to the performance that they
need, then they can take them through a disciplinary
procedure to dismiss. Now what we find is, you get to that
point, by and large, employers will offer a deal to take
them out* [a Compromise Agreement?] *yeah, rather than
sack them...*

(Union official)

Who does the bullying?

Teachers at all levels of responsibility in schools described
being bullied by another member of staff, usually someone in
a more senior position. For Primary teachers the perpetrator
was usually the Headteacher or Deputy Head; for Secondary
teachers it was more often the Deputy Head, Head of department
or member of the senior management team. These differences
reflect the different organisational structure and size of Primary
and Secondary schools.

The exercise of informal power, for example resulting from
'influential friendships', or from a long established teacher
bullying a new-comer to the school was much less common, but
it was seen in both Primary and Secondary schools:

*I went there as an Advanced Skills Teacher... it was very
clear that the Head and the Administrative Officer... had
a very close friendship, and the administrator seemed to
run the school... the administrator... would come into
your classroom and would say, 'What are you doing about*

this?' while you were teaching, and I'd say 'Hold on just a minute': 'Well your dinner money number's wrong.' And apparently she treated everybody like that... [My TA] witnessed three incidents where [she was]... extremely rude to me in front of the children, and she said... 'Why do you not turn round to that lady and say don't do this', and I tried to explain to her about the politics within the school. And she said, 'Well I'm very sorry but I'm certainly not going to put up with that'. She went to the Head complaining: she never returned to the classroom, she was asked to leave.

(Primary teacher)

Union officials and Senior Managers had come across similar examples:

It's not just bullying by the Head... I have had contact from teachers who have been scared of their TAs and things like that.

(Union official)

They may have the power to bully, but it's not necessarily, it doesn't have to be that hierarchical thing... I've seen Head bullied as well [Who by?] *by other members of staff.*

(Secondary Headteacher)

Environmental pressures

Our data, information about leadership changes, and the teachers' own descriptions, suggest that those being bullied may be working in particularly pressured environments. Many bullying problems began with the arrival of a new Headteacher, or a change in senior management.

All of our Primary teachers (24) had experienced a change of leadership prior to being bullied (14 had a new Headteacher and 10 were in a new school). Twelve of our (15) Secondary teachers also experienced a change of leadership prior to being bullied (totalling 36 of 39 respondents). For the Primary teachers with a new Headteacher it was often that Headteacher's first Headship (9 of 14 respondents).

> *Everything was fine... so then the new Head came in and that's really when the trouble and the problems began.*
>
> (Primary teacher)

For our Secondary teachers the bullying they described tended to come from a Head of department (HOD) or Senior Manager, but it was nevertheless frequently linked to leadership change.

> *I'd been there for years and years and I was a Head of year and everything was going along very nicely and I was going to apply for senior management and then we had a new [HOD]. She started bullying me, she just stopped speaking to me to start with, she used to do things to me; she used to be quite horrible. At first I thought it was nothing, just her being a bit moody. But it just carried on and on and eventually... she refused to speak to me or look at me at all.*
>
> (Secondary teacher)

Senior managers and Union officials often encountered, and recognised, new Headship as a problem, though not always one of bullying:

> *All new Heads make changes, and sometimes people perceive that as bullying and actually it's not. And we do have issues where Heads have worked with somebody*

for twenty years, failed to deal with some issues, and the new Head comes in and does deal with it, and that's not bullying...

(Union official)

I know of at least three [Headteachers] who do this sort of thing, and do it on purpose to get rid of staff that they actually prefer not to have... the first thing they decide to do, before they even walk in the door, is to get rid of the old staff because they want their own ones in, that they can then mould to the way they want the school... it's easily done... where do you go if your Head's doing it to you?

(Primary Headteacher)

Twenty-six teachers spoke about the fearful atmosphere within their school after the arrival of a new Headteacher, or on joining a new school, and some (13) talked about the pressures that everyone in the school was under.

The staffroom, you can tell the quality of the staff health, can't you, by the staff room, and it became such a quiet place; they weren't laughing, people weren't calling across to each other. It was a very nervous place to be, because they felt they were being watched.

(Secondary teacher)

...there is a lot of this going on: talking in classes with the door closed, and looking at who's going past. An awful lot: talking in cupboards, crying in cupboards.

(Primary teacher)

Relevant inspection reports (obtained for all but 2 schools) showed that although many were in some difficulties (13 'requiring Improvement', 5 'inadequate'), the remaining 21 schools were deemed 'good' or 'outstanding'. But the teachers' descriptions of the atmosphere of fear, and the pressure to maintain or improve their current inspection grades occurred across all the schools.

> [A new Head came] *then it started... a lot of bullying... not myself at the time, but other members of staff who felt they were under a lot of pressure to produce the goods, and she kept going round saying, 'Oh, this is a failing school. This is a failing school! I was selected to sort out this failing school'. Well actually it wasn't a failing school and people felt under pressure, I saw people crying in the corridors, people upset, it was a very difficult time.*
>
> (Primary teacher)

Inspection ratings undoubtedly put pressure on Heads to improve or maintain grades:

> *...the stress is coming very largely from Ofsted, obviously in combination with the government, and it's hard to know where the division is... this constant pressure... to prove that you are improving, that your standards are going up all the time... I do think that Heads are under the most enormous pressure, which means that then the pressure goes onto the Senior Management Team... down to the class teacher. They're having to improve results all the time... and I think that successive governments have created that... it's just gone up and up all the time. So the pressure is unhealthy.*
>
> (Union official)

Support for teachers

All the teachers talked about support, but there were very few examples of this being offered or provided within their schools.

Eventually it got to the point where I made a complaint to my line manager... Then we had some meetings... I don't think she knew how to deal with it actually. She didn't realise how serious it was... I think she hoped it would go away but it didn't. It was just getting worse so I complained again. So then I decided I would go to the Deputy Head... [who] thought it was just an argument and would pass over... I was getting more and more ill and eventually I went to the Head and made a formal complaint to the Head in writing and asked her to do something about it, and she told me at the time she'd sort it out etc. but she didn't and it just went on and on. And by then, for me, it was the final straw.

(Secondary teacher)

But there were some instances of support for our bullied teachers:

So, Senior Leadership managed to talk her down to one written warning. [The Senior Management Team were actually quite supportive of you?] *Very supportive, yes...* [Did you feel you got any support from any other member of staff while all this was happening?] *No, not really. I did try to get them to stand up and be witnesses to what she had done but everybody was too frightened of her.*

(Primary teacher)

Some Secondary teachers were able to get support from other members of staff, usually another teacher:

They both came out of there saying, 'How have you put up with being treated like that for so long?' They were shocked and one of them said to me, 'If you want to make a complaint about that I'll back you'. I think the other one said something similar, but they both said, 'you shouldn't be putting up with this, we will accompany you if you want to put in a complaint to somebody.'

(Secondary teacher)

In Primary schools any support available usually came from TAs rather than other teachers:

...there were people that I confided in, but everybody again, everybody had their own things going on as well, you know what I mean? My support was more [from the] support staff who'd helped me through.

(Primary teacher)

Lack of support led a number of teachers to talk about feeling isolated:

...the inspection was on the Tuesday or the Wednesday, so I remember actually doing the classroom on my own and no one helped me, and I'd never felt so lonely in my life, it was awful, it really was.

(Primary teacher)

...in school you are uniquely isolated in a way in your work, because you're confronted with the children all day long, you have little time to communicate with colleagues at all. When you do communicate with them it needs to be supportive, it needs to be productive, it needs to be constructive, and it needs to help you feel part of a team, because you are so worn down by the work itself. And none of that was there for years and years.

(Secondary teacher)

A good deal of support came from family and friends, the teaching Unions, Occupational Health (OH) services and the Education Support Partnership (formerly TSN). In many cases Headteachers, as legally required, referred teachers to OH, because the stress and anxiety of the bullying had made them ill. OH is generally independent from the LA and the schools, and tends to be very supportive despite teachers' initial concerns about being referred to them.

> *It was quite intimidating... I think it was the standard letter but there was a paragraph in it about if you don't attend and you don't let us know, I think it said something like, that you won't get your sickpay and it might affect, I can't remember exactly, but I found it very threatening, it was going to affect my sickpay and possibly affect my job...* [OH said] *'You are obviously not fit to be* [at school]... *You shouldn't be there... It's right that you are signed off'.*
> (Primary teacher)

Union advice was consistent regarding OH:

> *...always do it. They're there to help you; they're not there to help the Head... They give advice and the Head really, if they've got anything about them, should follow that advice.*
> (Union official)

> *Some people see OH as a management tool. But even if they're being used in that way, you know, we advise members to say right, tell them what the problem is, tell them what the impact is that it's having on you. Once it's out, once it's on record, the employer is very foolhardy to ignore what OH is saying.*
> (Union official)

Some teachers felt that their Union's support and advice was invaluable, while others were less satisfied:

I contacted the Union, they were a bit slow initially and they weren't particularly helpful.

(Primary teacher)

[What did the Union say?] *Oh they were brilliant.*

(Secondary teacher)

Union officials acknowledged that they are not always able to achieve what their member wants:

Sometimes... what a member wants is justice... they want the person to acknowledge that they've been bullied, they want them to know what they've put them through. And I can completely understand that, but actually... we might be able to get an agreement that they don't work with that person again, or... maybe a change of line manager, or a protocol for communication, or a Compromise Agreement to get them out of there. We may be able to do that, but we wouldn't always be able to get them the resolution that gives them a sense of personal satisfaction.

(Union official)

Most teachers who contacted Education Support Partnership (TSN) found them to be very helpful:

I actually had far more support from TSN [than from the Union], far more support, they were far more helpful, far more proactive, they listened, this sounds like an advert for them, but no, they were really good, and they got me through.

(Primary teacher)

> *I contacted TSN and they were very good and I did have a
> series of counselling sessions, which I thought had worked,
> but it's the continual drip, drip, drip.*
>
> (Primary teacher)

Family and friends were often mentioned as great sources of support:

> *I'm lucky.. I have had [my husband] all the time to support
> me... And I'm fortunate that my husband is so able, so
> that... I had him to say, 'Let's do this', and 'I'll do it for
> you'. Because if I were on my own I couldn't have done it.*
>
> (Secondary teacher)

> *I relied very heavily on my parents... I was going in in
> tears every day, I was ringing my Dad every day on the
> way to work, just to try and pluck up the courage to get in.*
>
> (Primary teacher)

Teacher ill-health

At the time of the interviews all the teachers who described themselves as bullied also described themselves as ill. They were not asked any direct questions about their health, but they all told us about health problems. Thirty eight described new mental health illness as a consequence of bullying (the remaining teacher had a disabling physical condition prior to the bullying which continued afterwards). Almost two-thirds described serious levels of depression, for example:

> *I was suicidal... I've been on antidepressants, I've been on
> beta blockers, I've had God knows how much counselling,
> CBT, just with the feeling that I was completely shafted,*

run roughshod over... by her.

(Primary teacher)

...the doctor kept saying I needed to take time off... After one year I got counselling for stress and depression, I didn't take [the] antidepressant tablets. I tried them, but I couldn't work properly when I was taking them. They made me woozy... and I didn't take time off but I just saw the doctor regularly.

(Secondary teacher)

A further 14 who had not mentioned depression also described combinations of work related stress and anxiety.

Stress-related mental health problems include: suicidal feelings, migraines, panic attacks, sleep problems, crying, difficulty going out, blood pressure, palpitations, panic attacks and balance problems[8]. A Primary teacher, speaking brokenly and in tears said, '*It's destroying me. It's led me to think of suicide*'. Another said of her doctor:

He had no hesitation at all, he just signed me off. He said 'no you're not fit to be going back'. Because I was, I mean for a while, it was physical symptoms really first, I was just aching all over, hurting physically, aching, constant headaches, I'd been under the hospital because I'd kept going dizzy, and they said it was something like a balance problem and everything. But when we got all the feedback... this balance problem can be stress induced. The physical effects, it got worse before it got better... the chest pains and breathing, all the anxiety more than anything.

(Primary teacher)

---

8   For more comprehensive details about the causes and symptoms of stress-related health problems and also for advice about how to manage them, see for example: Mind (2015) and Unison (2014).

I went home and carried on crying, and phoned in sick the next day and it was just a mess... I did go back to the doctor and was diagnosed with severe depression and severe anxiety. Symptoms such as extreme dizziness, in fact it was so severe that they tested me for other physical things in case it was something else... I hadn't seen it coming... It was sudden, it was like a switch. I've not been diagnosed with depression before.

(Secondary teacher)

Twenty seven of our teachers with post-bullying mental health problems had extended periods of sick-leave, but some were determined not to do so. Our Union officials recognised this behaviour and were concerned about it:

So you'll get people going into work when they really shouldn't be in, because they're too ill, which just increases the stress levels... people get into this vicious circle, and won't stay off because they might say I can't do the job, but I can't do the job because I'm ill, but if I stay off they're going say I can't do it', and it goes round and round and round.

(Union official)

They also said that they often feel obliged to advise members to take CAs that were offered, to avoid further damage to their health:

...quite often, we can't deal with it because we know that it's going to damage the individual member... sometimes you are saying to them: it might be in your best interests to leave the school. And that's just awful, as a trade Unionist... It's probably the best advice you can give in those circumstances, but it's terrible to have to do it.

(Union official)

Impact

Only 10 of our 39 teachers were actually teaching at the time of interview (5 were in the same school where the bullying had taken place and 5 were in new schools). Fifteen teachers were on long-term sick leave. Of the remaining 14, none of whom were teaching at the time, most said that they would never teach again (see Figs. 3 & 4 below)

> *It's finished my career. I don't think I'll ever teach again.*
>
> (Primary teacher)

> *It is unlikely that I will return to work in schools. The very thought of having to deal with anyone who could possibly act in the way that my previous Line Manager did is enough to keep me out. I love the teaching but have realised that my health and happiness means more to me and my family than anything else.*
>
> (Secondary teacher)

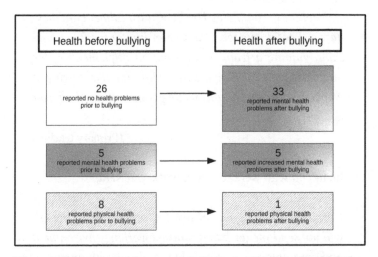

Figure. 3: Thirty nine teacher reports, at interview in 2012, of health before and after bullying

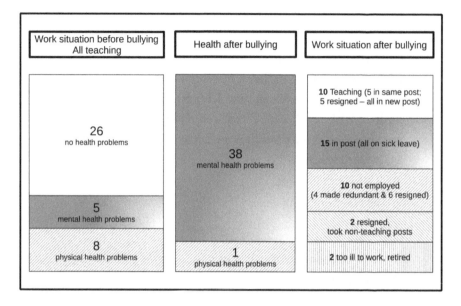

Figure 4: Thirty-nine teacher accounts of work situation in 2012 before and after bullying

One teacher now working in the training industry said:

> ...people have commented on how much calmer I am these days... I got a new job... as a co-ordinator for functional skills, guiding a team of assessors on implementing the qualification within apprenticeships. It's like having a whole new career and has really got me enthused all over again
>
> (Primary teacher)

Of the fifteen who were too ill to work, one said:

> I continue to be signed off sick (18 months now) my GP will not send me back to an unsafe working environment and my employers have failed to resolve the situation.
>
> (Primary teacher)

Of the 10 who continued to teach in schools, 6 had full-time posts (5 in the same school), and the remaining 4 were working as supply or part-time teachers in new schools. One Primary teacher bullied by CP and threats into resigning without a job said:

> *When I look at it now, if I try and look at it on the positive side, she did me a favour, because I've got a fantastic job, absolutely fantastic. I secured the position the final week of the Summer term, as I was leaving… it's a full-time job. It was temporary for one term until December but I proved myself within the first half term and they offered it me for the whole year… And I've been rated by LA reviews as good to outstanding.*
>
> (Primary teacher)

A Secondary teacher still working in the same school said:

> *She is 65 in May… It really sort of sucks the spirit out of me, and I get it back by trying to sort of keep in mind what's really important, like seeing all my grandchildren, who are 6, two 4 year olds and two 2year olds. So there's lots of balancing, positive balancing… when I didn't think anybody knew what was really happening, or couldn't really identify it myself, it was absolutely appalling. But now I can identify and, sort of, not quite give it back to where it's come from but I'm getting better at doing that. And of course I drink too much… A hundred and thirteen [days until she retires]. Trouble is she's never sick!*
>
> (Secondary teacher)

Another, now working part-time in the same school said:

> *Ill health got worse. I had migraines and panic attacks… Now I am part-time I am excluded from meetings because*

they are held on days when I'm not in… There is another observation due now and I am absolutely terrified because I can only do what I normally do and no support is being offered.

(Secondary teacher)

3.3

Reasons Offered by Teachers for the Bullying

Most of the reasons offered focused on the victim or the perpetrator's individual circumstances and/or on environmental factors. Teachers from Primary schools (but not Secondary schools) suggested that their age, their pay grade or mental health issues were possible reasons: *...no people are employing older people because we are expensive, the very reason that* [the Headteacher] *was getting rid of us.* (Primary teacher)

A Primary teacher with clinical depression, who had informed her Headteacher in writing said:

> *... she had always told me how expensive my insurance was... it was such a small school... only 80 children ... but 3 teachers there full time, including herself... so the school was over staffed... she was probably facing a redundancy situation, because none of us looked likely to leave... if one of us left she would be able to get in a NQT[9] or somebody in part time... I was an easy target... she knew there was a weakness there... she could see all that anxiety and stress was just under the surface and it didn't take much for me to go over the edge.*

> (Primary teacher)

---

9   Newly Qualified Teacher

Some thought the perpetrator might be feeling threatened, unable to cope with the stress of their job, or be lacking in experience or training for leadership:

> [What was behind it all?] *I think I intimidated her... I walked in there and I was confident, I was together. I'd got on with all the other members of staff. And she'd created this lovely little bubble for herself, and I came into it, and I threatened her.*
>
> (Primary teacher)

> *She was a very insecure woman... as I became more confident and I passed my NQT year you know, with flying colours and stuff, she started getting more and more bullying... she obviously felt threatened in some way... having thought about it, I think that the Head of Department was actually quite jealous of all the professional experience I had.*
>
> (Secondary teacher)

> *I just think that's how she dealt with things, so a panic mechanism. As she got more stressed she got rid of it by pushing it out there, and bullying other people.*
>
> (Secondary teacher)

Other reasons offered included the management system, school culture and external structures and pressures.

> *...because he was inadequate as a Head it was impacting ... further into the senior management level, and then very much so, through inadequacy really, on to the other members of staff. And that was definite bullying because people, the management, were frightened for their jobs, I think.*
>
> (Secondary teacher)

The system has failed – what she [the bully] *did wrong the system didn't deal with.*

(Primary teacher)

I do think stress put on her by the LA, by the possibility of Ofsted coming in, by the possibility of special measures. The progress is going down and down every year. I think she probably has an enormous amount of stress…

(Primary teacher)

3.4

Reasons Offered by Senior Managers and Union officials for the bullying

Senior Managers and Union officials came to similar conclusions. In response to our vignettes of the bullied teachers' experiences the great majority said similar things.

> *My experience as a class teacher, and as a Deputy Head, is that the culture... can be made or broken by the Head. But that in the same way, the Heads are subject to a huge amount of stress themselves, and I think one of the really difficult things as Head, as I've now discovered, is not just passing all that stress to your staff, and some Heads are better at it than others.*
>
> (Primary Headteacher)

> *...all of these external pressures, from government policy level, just filter down. And it goes on the Head's shoulders, he off-loads on to me... I hope I don't off-load onto other people... but then the pressures inevitably get transferred down.*
>
> (Secondary Deputy Head)

> *You don't know what pressure the Head's under, it doesn't excuse the behaviour... Sometimes it may be, if you've got a really good teacher, the Head actually feels intimidated and insecure, by having somebody who is very good.*

And they'd perhaps rather have somebody who doesn't challenge them as much.

(Union official)

The stresses and strains that schools and their managers are subject to in the current educational environment are issues that we will return to in our final chapter. However, to conclude Chapter 3 we outline below some of the suggestions our respondents made regarding ways to challenge and change the bullying behaviours they reported having experienced in their schools.

3.5

Ways Forward

We asked what could be done to create an educational workplace that might mitigate bullying. Almost all our respondents had suggestions, the most common being:

- An independent body to mediate or intervene if needed, but definitely **not** Ofsted or Governors.
- Collective action.
- Management training and communications.

> *I think it would be better if... there was somebody independent... in a position of some authority... there aren't enough impartial people... It could be someone seconded up for that post. Like there is someone for Child Protection.*
>
> (Secondary teacher)

> *...I think the single biggest thing that's missing from all schools is somebody independent... because... everything that goes through the school goes through the Head... when a teacher's going to be dismissed, or suspended, the teacher should be referred to a panel of completely independent lay people.*
>
> (Primary teacher)

There was a strong feeling that approaching the governors would not be helpful because they were not really independent of the Headteacher, who was often cited as the bully.

> *I think that the Chair of Governors and the governors usually agree with what the Head says.*
>
> (Secondary teacher)

> *So in theory yes, if you've got a problem with your Head you should go to the governors, but also in practise most governors are going to back the Head.*
>
> (Primary Headteacher)

> *By and large a Head will have the governing body in his or her pocket, if they've got any sense, and so you... go into a disciplinary hearing and the decision has already been made before you walk through the door, regardless of the strength of your case.*
>
> (Union official)

Ten teachers felt that collective action might be effective, but that fellow staff were too frightened to help:

> *I mean members of staff have seen what has happened at the school but they are too scared to do anything about it. I've said to them, 'Let's go to the Union as a group'... and [R] and I were the only two... because all the rest backed out.*
>
> (Primary teacher)

> *[The other teachers] told me that they didn't want to do anything that would upset her, and when I was off sick my Union approached them and asked if they wanted to join in with the grievance and they didn't. They said no because they were too frightened and there'd be repercussions.*
>
> (Primary teacher)

The Union officials understood teachers' fears but still believed that taking collective action was an effective way forward.

I can understand why some individuals don't want to do that because they don't want to be identified... Heads pick members off, go to the weakest... which then gets them to withdraw or not sign up to it... Collective action is always much more powerful than individuals.

(Union official)

...if we can get to deal with it collectively on behalf of members, we know it's going to work... it has to be a significant number. Because if you can say to the Head, the governors, or an independent investigation, we've got, as we did in the very first school that we tried this in, we had 37 members out of a staff of 70-odd [complaining]. *This is massively significant... And that's where you get the weight of evidence to actually deal with it.*

(Union official)

Many teachers felt that Senior Managers should have better training and better communication skills:

[They] *actually need to listen to people. And they need to take it seriously when someone says they're being bullied... so I think maybe it is down to training really... they don't seem to be very good communicators... so I suppose it's about communication and training.*

(Secondary teacher)

Some Senior Managers felt that bullying issues were not sufficiently covered during their training course and that while some Heads would seek the necessary training others would not.

I think personnel issues are very difficult to deal with and

> *there are some people who are in management positions*
> *who either haven't been trained, or they haven't got their*
> *own personal set of skills to be able to deal with these*
> *things, or they find it quite intimidating.*
>
> (Primary Headteacher)

The Union officials were well aware of the pressures on Senior Managers in schools and the support they needed:

> *We hold briefings and events for school leaders... we*
> *recognise... there are some issues that are very specific to*
> *Heads, and their personal and professional development is*
> *just as important as is that of the staff... this is something*
> *that we think should be provided nationally, you know, for*
> *all senior leaders.*
>
> (Union official)

They also talked in detail about what could be done to change a bullying situation, and all were in agreement that it was important to try to work with the schools:

> *...what we're trying to do, invariably, is not to litigate*
> *against schools, but to get in there, and to work with*
> *them... it's usually more productive if you don't lodge a*
> *grievance but you still engage in the discussion, to seek to*
> *reform it, to resolve it informally, if that's possible.*
>
> (Union official)

An important early step for teachers with grievances was to involve the Union, who could help, advise, and be present in any meetings. There was also agreement that keeping a written (or e-mail) record of what had happened was vitally important because often it was the only source of evidence:

...that way we can say, 'Look. This is our record of things that have been happening'. And once the Head, or someone, can see this it kind of makes them sit up and think, 'Wow. I need to back off a bit here. This person's keeping a record'. And often that can change the relationship.

(Union official)

...it's always useful to have some record or some evidence, so one of the basic things we do is, we say, keep a log or write down a list of things... asking them to put something in writing... just seek explanations of things, you know, maybe: 'you were disappointed to know that you weren't included in this meeting, it could have been useful to you', 'is there an explanation for it'... because someone could turn round and say: well why didn't you say something at the time. And that is really, really difficult...

(Union official)

Independent arbitration for teachers feeling bullied or threatened, plus better training and support for Senior Managers, were key issues for our teachers regarding 'what could be done'. For our Union officials, good record keeping of events, and working with schools and their managers, alongside collective action by their members, were their main suggestions. While the teachers recognised that collective action could be an effective way forward they were largely unconvinced that colleagues would 'stand up and be counted' given the climate of fear they experienced and expressed.

3.6

Summary and Conclusions

Despite their unique individual stories and differences we found a number of notable commonalities amongst our teachers: almost all (32 of 39) had experienced a recent change of leadership or Headship, and all but one reported deteriorating mental health as a result of the bullying they experienced.

There were also many descriptions of a fearful environment, often internal to the school, or ascribed to external pressures by teachers, Senior Managers and Union officials, plus suggestions that some Heads may be using CPs to remove staff that they regard as potential threats.

Collective action was clearly an issue for our Union officials and it was their recommended way forward. It was also recognised as a possible way forward by a number of teachers, but with reservations, and this will be explored further in the following stories, responses and commentaries in Section 2, and in our concluding chapter, in relation both to the data presented here, and the context, literature and research on workplace bullying presented in Section 1.

The teachers' narratives that follow are derived from, and more formally evidenced in, the research data presented above. They allow us to give greater voice to the teachers' (and Senior Managers' and Union officials') real-life experiences of bullying in the educational workplace whilst at the same time maintaining the essential and promised confidentiality regarding individual respondent's unique experiences and their schools identities.

SECTION TWO

What the teachers, managers and unions said

Introduction

Section two aims to show in detail what our volunteer teachers, Senior Managers and Union officials said, thought and felt about bullying, using their own words as far as possible, while still retaining their anonymity. Each of the stories, responses and commentaries presented here are derived from, and more formally evidenced in, the research data presented in Chapter 3.

To ensure individual anonymity we use pseudonyms and fictionalised settings for the teachers' stories in Chapter 4. Each story is based in the main on one individual teacher's interview. But since a number of teachers described the same type of bully and bullying, some from within the same school, we have included some of their words where they add substance. In every story the setting corresponds to that of the teachers whose stories we tell.

In Chapter 5, the Senior Managers' responses come entirely from our interviews with them. Each Manager was given two or three comprehensive and detailed narratives (vignettes) from individual teachers who had been bullied. These accounts were from teachers who worked in the same sector as the Senior Manager so inevitably not all Managers read the same accounts. Some of these accounts represent the combined opinions of a number of Managers with similar views about the same topic while others are based entirely on a single Manager's responses.

In our interviews with Union officials a number of common

themes emerged and there was much agreement between the four different unions and their seven representatives. Thus, the commentaries in Chapter 6 are presented as single threads, each one focusing on an issue of importance to Union officials.

4

THE TEACHERS' STORIES

4.1

Jenny's story: the party

My name is Jenny. I was bullied by my Headteacher. I started teaching there as an NQT and the Headteacher offered me a permanent post as a full-time class teacher for the following year. But then a new Headteacher took over. She seemed okay at first, she was making quite a lot of changes but it seemed okay until her second term at the school. I am not at that school now but a recent event reminded me of what happened then.

The final straw was when she summoned me to a meeting saying: 'In my opinion you are not a teacher; you've adopted the role of a Level 3 Teaching Assistant. The children in your classes aren't learning this year.' And she attacked me for behaviour management in assemblies, but now I was angry because I knew this wasn't true, so I answered her back, telling her that as a peripatetic teacher I rarely took the children to assemblies. It was just blatant lies. But what do you do? She ended the meeting by saying that if progress and development hadn't been made by Christmas, Capability Proceedings would begin. At this point I just stayed quiet; there was no point in me talking; whatever I said didn't really matter.

Then I contacted my Union. They advised me to make a formal complaint of bullying. But I was a young teacher up against the Head who, for whatever reason, had decided that she didn't want me at the school and had taken action to force me out, to literally constructively dismiss me. I didn't want to jeopardise my future career by being known as the one who gets the Union involved. I knew that's what you had to do, but in your head it's more difficult. Later in my career perhaps I might have done it. But not at that stage with her – she could charm the birds off the trees. I felt the only course I could take was to hand in my notice.

At that time I thought I would never go back but Barbara, my best friend, phoned to invite me. Marie, my old Head of Foundation, was retiring and there was going to be a party for her at school. The thought of going back there made me feel sick. But Barbara was insistent: 'Marie was a wonderful support, even though in the end she could do nothing to help you. You should be there. I'll come and meet you in the car park.'

I had to ask: 'Will Mrs Fisher be there?' Even her name made me feel tense and jittery.

'Don't worry, she left last year, after a really bad Ofsted, and she's not likely to show her face again now.' So I agreed.

It was a large school, on the outskirts of the city, in quite a deprived area. Most families were on benefits. As I pulled into the car park the memories came flooding back. I could see the windows of my first classroom; that year as a newly qualified teacher was a happy one. I had a fantastic year with every observation positive, and it was a lovely place to work, with friendly, happy people. The children were difficult but I enjoyed the challenge of it all and I got lots of support until the new Head came.

I began to feel really panicky. Barbara was there in the car park as she had promised. As we walked in together the memories came flooding back: the one-off, constant, unsupported comments, the sleepless nights, the undermining of my confidence.

It had started just a term into her Headship. There had been no observations beforehand; it came out of the blue. I'd sent 7 children from my class to our behaviour mentor because of their extreme rudeness to me. The next day the Head came into my room at 8:25am and closed the door, saying she wanted to talk to me; she told me I was a rubbish teacher. I should think about looking for another school, another job, maybe teaching wasn't the career for me, or maybe this wasn't the school for me. But if I did apply for another job she would not be able to give me a good reference. Then she left, saying 'Think about what I said. I'll talk to you in a few days.' She left, my room with 5 minutes to go until school started; I only just managed to hold myself together to teach the kids.

Then, for a while, it was just lots of little things, whenever I was on my own with her. I found myself hiding in cupboards, so that she wouldn't be able to come and criticise me. And I would think – I'm 27, why am I standing here in the dark not wanting her to know I'm here? My health and confidence suffered. She threatened me with Capability without evidence, and without saying what I needed to develop or what targets to aim for.

She created an environment of intimidation, bullying and harassment, and at the end of that year at least three teachers left, because of the same situation. They couldn't handle it any more; they wanted to leave. But I was being stubborn, thinking – she can't make me leave! I will stay! That probably backfired because I was the only one left that she wanted to get rid of, so everything focused on me. I got moved to a peripatetic role to cover Foundation for 2 days, Year 1 for 1 day and PPA[10] cover for teachers from Years 1, 2 and 3 the rest of the time. I had a shared responsibility with the class teachers when I looked after their classes but no ownership of them. I was confused. I didn't understand. Was she doing this to push me out? I left that Christmas, a year after it all started; I felt so worthless.

I didn't really do much for months, but eventually I did a day's supply work at another school. They kept asking for me again. The supply days extended and extended: they were really happy with me. It was a very small school with kind and supportive people, my confidence was pretty much back and I actually enjoyed going to work. When I left them my confidence was back to where it had been before 'Her'.

---

10   Planning and Preparation Allowance

I got a job in Foundation Stage (my preferred age group) in an inner city school. My old, bullying, Head had always told me she didn't believe inner city schools were the right place for me so I was a little worried when I started. But she was wrong! I loved it, everything was so positive, the Foundation Stage team I worked with thought I was amazing, and the Head agreed (something I still find hard to hear); I never had less than good for any observations. I still found it difficult to be observed as I always expected the worse, but it got easier. I'm in my second year there, and the Head has been so positive about me she has made me a member of the management team.

Even though Mrs Fisher wasn't at the party it was still the place where it had all happened, and it did bring back horrible memories. But now it's over and I'm so glad that Barbara insisted I came. Now I will never have to worry about bumping into old members of staff and wondering what to say. I felt confident and happy as I walked away back to my car.

Jenny recently told us: My job is hard and does sometimes stress me out but most jobs are like that. I'm just glad that it's all for the right reasons. I am so glad that when I was told *'teaching isn't the right job for you'* that I didn't listen. It was the job I had always wanted to do and the job I still want to do.

4.2

Jo's story: it just got worse and worse

Jo is in her early 40s, has been a teacher for 22 years, and is currently on sick leave from the girls' comprehensive school where she has worked since 1994, and where she had been a Head of Year in KS4 when the present Headteacher arrived in September 2005. Everything was going along very nicely and she was about to apply for a senior management post. Her HOD retired and in September 2003 a new person, Erica, was appointed. The small department had 4 members of staff: Erica (new HOD), Ann (Deputy HOD), Jo and Sandy.

The bullying began in March 2004, when Erica just stopped speaking to me. At first I thought it was nothing, just Erica being a bit moody. Then she started to do cruel, horrible things to me. She would accuse me of things in front of other staff, she ignored me in front of the pupils, she refused to allow me to go on any training, or to organise any training for me, and she made it difficult for me to do my job.

It got progressively worse, until I hated being in the department. I started to keep notes of what happened and dates when things happened. By the Autumn term things had got to the point where I made a complaint to my line manager, Heather, who arranged a meeting with me and Erica together, but Heather was her line manager too.

In the meeting Erica said that I had brought the department into disrepute, that I gave a bad impression of the department around the school, that the only reason her own year groups were successful was because there was no-one like me in them, and she said that she had no professional responsibility to speak to me. When I asked why she wouldn't allow me to go on training courses Erica said that I wasn't entitled to any professional development. I asked her to tell Heather what it was that I had done wrong, but Erica refused to say anything or even to look at me. Heather made no comment and at the end of the meeting said, 'Well I think that's sorted things out now.' Afterwards I spoke to Heather and asked why she had let Erica get away with saying these things. Heather said that I was the stronger party, but I felt that she didn't realise how serious the situation was, and also that she just didn't know how to deal with it.

I hoped the problem would go away but it just got worse, so a month later I complained again. This time I went to Pam, one of the Deputy Heads, who was very well respected in the school. Pam promised to deal with it, but still nothing changed. I felt very let down. Much later, when I returned to school after a long sickness absence, I asked Pam why she hadn't done anything about Erica's behaviour. Pam told me that she had made Erica sit at a computer and look up all the training and professional development courses, to pick out and make a list of ones for me, and to make sure I knew about them and was able to go on them. But Erica never did. Had I known, I could have done something about it at the time.

I was getting more and more ill. Eventually I made a formal complaint in writing to the Head, asking to have something done about Erica's behaviour. She told me she'd sort it out, but nothing changed, and the bullying continued.

Then one day in December 2004, I finally broke down completely. I remember crying all the way home in the car after school. I went to my doctor, who referred me to a psychiatrist. I went back to work after a few days, but I wasn't at all well. Although I'd not been away from school for very long the Head referred me to

Occupational Health, saying that I was experiencing psychiatric problems which she believed were school related. My appointment was for the first day of the Spring term.

Some teacher training students were to be in the department during the Spring term, so, before Christmas, I asked Erica whether there was to be an observation period or whether the students would be teaching immediately. She told me they would be teaching immediately. So, on the first day of term a student was to teach my first lesson, and after that I was due at Occupational Health. I asked to have a look at the student's lesson plan, but the student said there was an observation period so she wasn't teaching. When I asked Erica, she said, 'Oh yes, we changed it.' So, despite not having planned it, I taught the lesson with the student watching. Then I went to see the Occupational Health doctor and she said that I had to have time off work.

While I was off work I took out a grievance against Erica. Then the Head got in touch, saying that Erica had handed in her notice, and asking did I still want to go ahead with the grievance. I said yes. The schools Effectiveness Inspector heard the grievance. A number of witnesses were interviewed, including Ann, the Deputy HOD, who told how miserable she was working with Erica, and Heather told them that she found the whole situation impossible because she was line manager for both of us. In June 2005 I received a letter saying that the grievance had failed on the grounds that the Union's definition of bullying had not satisfactorily been proved. But they didn't take account of the cumulative nature of bullying, the collective nature of small events, because bullying isn't one big thing, it's a collection of small things. I didn't appeal because by then both the Head and Erica were leaving the school, and if I did appeal I'd have to go through it all again.

I felt well enough to go back to work by the end of the Summer holidays but, because the new Head felt I was emotionally fragile, I wasn't Head of Year, even though I kept my HOY timetable. In the extra time I did mentoring to Y11 students, but I couldn't manage professional development days or my performance management lesson observations because I would start crying.

By the end of 2006 I was well enough to go back to being HOY. I had a new line manager who I got on with really well. But I continued to have mental health problems, and needed a lot of support with my performance management. I had an agreement that the Head would do my observations, and that I could ask her to leave at any time if I became upset. Everything went OK until one day when I had a lesson observation due and the Head was unable to come. Instead she sent Anita, one of Erica's closest friends, to observe me and everything went wrong: the class were late arriving, I ended up just losing it with Anita, and I was sent home again. I've not been back since, and I don't think I will ever be fit enough to work full time again.

I've been ill ever since that bullying. I've never recovered. Erica went off to another school with no stain on her record, and I'm left like this. There's no question that I would ever be a HOY again, or a Senior Manager, that I would ever be anything. I just seem to be going lower and lower in the ranks of what I can achieve. The Head is very supportive because she knows what went on, even though she wasn't there at the time. But she is in two camps: on the one hand she is very supportive, but on the other hand she wants to get rid of me because I'm expensive. And the reason I'm expensive is that I used to do a really good job.

Jo recently told us: I don't earn much money unfortunately, and I don't have a pension any more. I still suffer from anxiety and can't do a lot work-wise. I have got used to being an underachiever now. I will never go back to teaching in a school. The teacher who bullied me is still doing well as a Head of Faculty at her new school. Good salary and pension as well I suppose. The good thing about having left teaching is that now I have peace of mind – most of the time!

4.3

Pauline's story: old and experienced means expensive too!

Pauline is a bullied teacher, one of four out of a total of six at Northminster Primary school. Their new Headteacher caused them unnecessary stress, accused them of incompetence with no evidence, drove them into illness, depression and eventually resignation from the school, which was convenient because Northminster had a big budget deficit and was in need of either redundancies or 'wastage'. Pauline was wary of the new Headteacher right from the start. He was fresh out of Industry, middle-aged, had been in Management all his life, and had only been teaching for a few years when he came to them as Headteacher.

He was inexperienced, the only applicant, and was given the post temporarily in the November, and then had to re-apply for the job in March. So he had to show he was going to do something in that short period of time. And that's what he set out to do. It was clear that he was going to make a lot of changes and that he wasn't going to ask anybody if they agreed with him. Just a few years experience, and there was Jean with her 33 years, Michael with his 37, and me with my 25 and the others – everybody was experienced – which, as it turned out, was unfortunate for us oldies, because it meant that we were quite expensive to employ.

He sent round memos about untidy classrooms, and displays that were too celebratory, telling us to clear our shelves of children's work. He set impossible deadlines and gave us endless menial and pointless tasks to do. His planning sheets had to be in a specific format, but everyone had trouble with them. It took hours and hours, and although there were lots of planning materials available we weren't allowed to use them. He scribbled all over my plans. I felt victimised, intimidated, bullied and harassed and it was just at the time when redundancies were needed because of the school's big budget deficit. During a year of bullying he made me feel that my whole career was tarnished. He had no competence or credibility as a teacher, or as a judge of me and my career, but the insidious effect of his repeated bullying left me in pieces. I was off sick with depression, anxiety and stress for a long time before eventually I took out a grievance against him. The Governors said that the Head had acted professionally at all times and there was nothing to answer. Then I took it to appeal. But they said he had apologised for getting the wording of the disciplinary wrong and so he had nothing to answer. I lost the appeal but I had resigned by then.

The others could see what was happening to me but were afraid to speak out, worried about their own positions, really. Governors focused on the issue of staff cuts and budgets, and turned a blind eye to any complaints against Mr Frost. Their minutes of meetings showed that he was looking at senior teachers' salaries, looking at getting rid and reducing costs. When I resigned my teaching hours were given to the Teaching Assistant, saving the school quite a lot of money. Eventually Jenny, Michael and Jean also left Northminster, after long absences on sick leave, and for similar reasons to mine. We were all surprised when Mr Frost suddenly left – in the middle of Summer – without giving any notice, obviously under some sort of cloud or something. It was then that we decided to write to the local paper.

Northminster Echo: 26th August 2012

Older teachers bullied out to reduce costs at local school.

Four of the six teachers at Northminster Primary school have resigned and written to the Echo claiming that they were bullied by the headteacher Mr Frost, who resigned last week and left without giving any notice. One had taken out a grievance against the head alleging that she had been bullied. The union got involved and advised all four teachers to raise a collective grievance, but at that time the other 3 were scared of losing their jobs and getting a bad reference.

All four teachers are very experienced, each having taught for over 20 years with no major health problems, yet all had developed symptoms of stress and depression within 6 months of the arrival of the new head teacher, resulting in long-term sick leave and pupils being taught by inexperienced supply teachers.

Mr Frost joined the school only two years ago. When he took over, Northminster had just been graded by Ofsted as an 'improving school with some good features'. Minutes from the Governing Body meeting in Mr Frost's first term show that the school had an operating deficit of nearly £40,000, and this was expected to continue into the following year. One year later, with 4 experienced teachers on long-term sick leave, Governors' minutes recorded that they must reduce the predicted deficit by decreasing staffing costs. It was agreed to recommend making one teacher redundant (unless a resignation is received from a member of teaching staff)."

school year in a couple of weeks time. Ofsted has also recently downgraded the school to 'in need of improvement', noting that many staff are either new to their post or lack sufficient experience and expertise. Mr Frost's Deputy has stepped up to take on the roll of acting head.

In their open letter to the Echo the four teachers stated:

Mr Frost's conduct towards us as experienced teachers at the top of the salary scale suggests that he had an agenda, which included getting rid of expensive teaching staff by whatever means, in order to reduce Northminster's budget deficit, in some cases replacing qualified teachers with teaching assistants. As a scheme it failed because the school's budget reports show that Mr Frost spent £60,000 on supply teachers' salaries in just one year!

> *He calculated "savings" in terms of salaries, against potential teacher resignations, and told the Governors that "the major barrier to the educational progress of the children was staff absence".*
>
> *It was Mr Frost's actions that created the gaps in staffing. He never undertook any teaching himself, no matter how short of staff the school was. Instead he employed supply teachers and deployed teaching assistants (with no planning provided) to cover classes.*
>
> *Mr Frost left this month, without notice, but no action has been taken against him for breaching the terms and conditions of his employment contract. We consistently called for a closed investigation, in order to avoid bringing adverse publicity to the school, but now it is too late for that.*
>
> Our reporter investigated the school and discovered that Mr Frost had indeed resigned and left the school without working his notice, leaving Northminster with a huge budget deficit, a falling roll, the loss of 4 experienced teachers, and without a head teacher for the start of the new year.

Pauline recently told us: Northminster, post Mr Frost, is still struggling and doesn't appear to be anywhere near a recovery. We, *'the ousted'*, have turned our lives around relatively quickly, but the toll on us, health-wise, was significant. I'm happy with my lot, but glad to be out of teaching (with all the pressure I witnessed being heaped on schools), as it had provided me with lots of other opportunities – although, obviously, I wouldn't have chosen to be bullied. The Local Authority has repeatedly refused requests to discuss the case, and most parents are probably still unaware of the lies and distortions and the unjust treatment meted out to teachers at the school. We feel that the whole matter has been swept under the carpet by those responsible for Mr Frost's appointment, and their subsequent support of him as Headteacher. It was a source of such pain to all of us who fell victim to him that we are reluctant to press for the reopening of old wounds.

4.4

Debbie's story: depression *is* an illness

Debbie is an experienced Modern Foreign Languages (MFL) Secondary school teacher who had been teaching in the same school for 8 years. She suffered from clinical depression, and had informed the school about this verbally and in writing long before she became pregnant for the first time.

I was looking forward to the birth of my first child. I'd always wanted to be a mum. My husband and I were delighted, but we were both worried because I miscarried in April 2009: I had to take a week off back then. In late May 2009 I found out I was pregnant again. From then on I was just in fear of going to school, of going to work. I was feeling very worried because the pregnancy came along so soon after the miscarriage, and I was scared of what was going to happen. Then in the Autumn term my blood pressure was up, and I was on the way to pre-eclampsia.

It was early December when the HOD came into my classroom and shouted at me, in front of all the students, because those folding walls between our classrooms hadn't been put back properly, and a pupil was spying through it and calling out. She wanted a word with me after school, and she was really, really nasty, saying 'Pull yourself together.' I felt really down, because I was exhausted. And the next day my blood pressure was so high, I was seriously ill, and I ended up in hospital. We got through Christmas but I was still very ill, to the point where I couldn't even open my eyes because the headaches were so bad. Phoebe was born three weeks early.

*When she arrived I was not coping mentally, not quite where
I should have been, and then it all fell apart. I was in the dark
depths of postnatal depression and I didn't think I'd ever recover. It
took a long time for my blood pressure to go back to normal. Then
I was on maternity leave for a year, and just beginning to get over
the depression when I went back.*

*My mental health had been pretty good for most of my time
teaching, but I did get bouts of depression, and I'd always been
honest about it with the school. Mrs Parker, the previous HOD
knew and understood, and she gave me support whenever I needed
it: if I'd been off for a while, for my first term back, she made sure
I had a light timetable, and that I would be teaching my main
language, German, most of the time.*

*When I went back I asked to go part-time, 4 days a week.
They agreed but gave me a horrible timetable, mostly bottom
sets, and I wasn't teaching much German. I had some problems
in observations, because things had changed during the year I'd
been away, and nobody had told me about the different teaching
approaches expected, like the Planners and Target Sheets. A new
Head had arrived just before I went on maternity leave, but all the
changes had come in while I was away, so I had no idea how they
wanted things taught. We were supposed to have the Planner to
hand, in case Senior Management did learning walks, and these
had almost tripled. I had an observation two weeks after I came
back from maternity leave, and I got an inadequate. It was just
awful, so I said, 'Right. Come in and observe me again, I'll show
you.' And I did. I got a satisfactory and thought well, fair enough,
I can improve on that. I can take constructive criticism because
I love my job, you know, I absolutely love it, but not being told
all the time that 'Oh you're really bad at teaching.' There was no
constructive feedback, no development time.*

*I remember, it was the beginning of March 2011. I'd had three
observations by then, and the HOD had a mentor meeting with
me. She was really horrible, and had this long list of very petty*

things. I was still only getting satisfactory in my lessons, and she said, 'It's a very shaky start.' That was it, I had a breakdown.

The Crisis Team psychiatric nurse and my doctor said I needed help, that I needed to take time off school, and they doubled the dose of my antidepressants. They kept saying, 'You need time off,' but I couldn't take any time off, that was the last thing I could do. I was too scared to take time off.

So I went back, and the HOD did another learning walk, me with another bottom set, and she came in and took over the lesson really. She moved all the students around, because I'd put some on the ends of rows just to stop them chattering, so they could get on with their work. But she moved them back, so it disrupted everything. It was totally undermining. It's not easy when you've got a bottom set with 30-odd kids, and you've got more than a handful that should be in a little access group or something, which they'd got rid of because of the budget problems. Later there was an announcement, saying that they needed people to cut their hours because of the school budget. I decided to go from 4 days to 3, which was a really good decision. Then it was the Summer holiday and that helped a bit. I was starting to feel better.

The next term I had lots of learning walks. I got an email from the HOD, saying that she was going to observe me again in two weeks, and this was the third time in one half-term. That was it, I got onto the Union and they were brilliant. They were concerned that I was having a third observation, and they told the Personnel Manager that I should not have any more observations until I'd seen OH. The Union rep came with me to OH, which was very good. But when we went in I just broke down. I said 'I've got depression. I've been trying to carry on'. They said, 'More time in-between observations would help, and having these extra observations is just ridiculous,' and they sent a massive long list of stuff in their report to the Head.

Suddenly the Head got involved. She called me to a meeting. The Personnel Manager was there taking notes but nobody from my department. She said she was putting me on informal Capability because she had serious concerns. I got very upset that day. She knew that I was suffering from this depression illness, that it was recurring, and that I was honest about it, but they wanted to get rid of somebody, so...

I was very stressed, feeling sick and getting headaches all the time. My doctor signed me off again. That was the 10th of November 2011, I remember it vividly. I was sent back to OH, and they told me that their first report had stated, 'No observations, just for a few weeks, to help her recovery.' But they said that the school had written back saying, 'Can you please take out the bit about observations because we will not make that adjustment.' The Union said it was discrimination, because the Head hadn't made any reasonable adjustments, and that it sounded like harassment. They wrote to the Head saying I would be covered by the Equalities Act 2010, because the school knew that I'd got depression, and that after you've had a breakdown and things, they should have done something to help me. After that I was off sick again. It went to Regional Office with the Union, and we began putting in a grievance against the Head and Head of Department.

I'm pleased to say that I have moved on a lot since that nightmare. I attended a meeting at the school with my Union rep as it reached regional level and the Head knew she had no chance of winning this one. Therefore, I called the shots and said I am not going back, but I'm not resigning either, I would see them in court, and I managed to get a Compromise Agreement with a surprisingly glowing reference which, as my Union rep told me, is highly unusual!

Later that year I was headhunted by a private tuition company, and now I am a tutor for them and I've helped expand their courses. Online work is great and I meet people from around the world. Recently I was offered work with the National Extension College too!

Debbie recently told us: she now runs her own business and it is thriving. She can work from home, teaches people of all ages, levels and languages, and is doing so well her business even has a waiting list! She said that it was exactly 3 years ago that she was called into the Headteacher's office and put on Capability. Since then she had heard that Ofsted said the department's standard of teaching was inadequate, that the results have been bad, there had been a high turnover of teachers in MFL and that the school has been in trouble again for discrimination. She said, 'I am so glad I'm not there!'

4.5

Emma's story: you can't win

Emma, a Primary school teacher in her mid 30s, had been teaching for 14 years. After 10 years in her previous school, where she had done a lot of ICT teaching, with lessons across every year group and with other schools, she applied for and got a job in a new school, one which allowed her an afternoon out each week to do ICT consultancy for the LA. Her new school was in a 'leafy area' and attainment levels were quite high, while her previous experience had always been in much more challenging schools.

After my first 14 years I could say 'So far so good', and in Ofsted-Speak 'Good to Outstanding'. I loved my work, I loved the kids, but it was time to move on: a new school, a new job and a move up the ladder. It looked perfect and the Head was so nice at the interview. But almost immediately I could tell that something wasn't quite right – an atmosphere, a staffroom where everyone is being careful what they say, walking on eggshells, afraid to speak in case 'she' overheard. At a staff meeting the Head said, 'Has anybody got an idea?', and no-one spoke. I said something and she replied, 'Oh, don't be ridiculous.' Everybody else was thinking 'Don't say anything, just shut up and agree with her.' At my first lesson observation with the Head she graded me 'satisfactory', despite the wording of each section saying 'good'.

It was a horrendous first year, I hated every second of it. Three terms of put-downs and humiliations by the Head; endless unannounced observations where she just turned up, randomly, and picked holes in everything I did, making me increasingly nervous, affecting my confidence. She said, repeatedly, that I was too expensive, not upholding discipline, not performing as well as others. I tried to adjust to the fact that I was just not a very good teacher anymore.

In September, the start of my second year there, I'm trying to be upbeat, positive, cheerful, and refusing to let it get me down. It looked OK! At my performance management meeting she said I'd met all my targets, nothing negative, and I felt reassured. Ofsted came and it was fine; I got 'Good to Outstanding' (as did all the other teachers). But it still didn't feel right, there was so much unpleasantness going on.

After a budget meeting she came into the staffroom and said, 'The budget's been cut by £20,000. We're probably going to have to lose staff.' The atmosphere in the staffroom was horrible, everyone was thinking, 'Will it be me?' My salary was about £20,000 more than that of an NQT! Then I got her feedback from the performance management meeting. I'd met the targets but she had added some really nasty comments: I've not supported whole school initiatives; I've refused to maintain the school's international link. Not true, and I had the evidence to prove it! But I was extremely upset by her comments and the unexpected nature of them. A senior member of staff warned me not to challenge her as it would 'only make things worse'. I tried to put it behind me and carry on but I felt very unsure of my position. Half-term holiday came and went in misery.

Two weeks before the end of term, and without warning, she sent a message: 'In my office in 5 minutes.' I didn't know what it was about. She said, 'I have concerns', and then she listed the most ridiculous things, but she had no evidence, none of it was true. 'She said, I intend to take formal proceedings if these things don't improve.' I asked, 'How can I improve on things that I am already doing?' And I made the mistake of adding 'And whatever I do, it won't be good enough for you.' She replied, 'Then you're not good enough for the school.' She said, 'If you choose to resign now you'll get a good reference. If you don't then I'll take Formal Proceedings and that will go on your reference.' There was no mention of any support for the issues she raised, assuming they were genuine. I tried to discuss it further but she said she wasn't interested in talking around in circles, and told me to leave the office. I don't remember much more of that day. I got through to the afternoon and I remember standing in front of the class, looking at the children and thinking, 'I don't care. I just don't care anymore.'

That term, every day, I came home crying. I was drinking more than was good for me, just to cope with it all, feeling sick, dreading going into work. I couldn't carry on like this. In the middle of the night I woke up with palpitations. I tried to go back to sleep, but by the time I got up I was shaking, not the sort of shaking, like when you're really cold, but my whole body. When I got out of the shower I just crumpled to the floor. I wasn't in pain or anything, but I just couldn't move, I was crying, and it was as if someone had just pulled all my bones out. I saw the doctor; she checked my blood pressure and it was really high. I broke down completely. She prescribed a multitude of medications, and said, 'I'm signing you off. You cannot go into work like this'.

The Union said I could take a grievance against the Head. I have the evidence, but no employer is going to want somebody who takes out grievances. The Union said I could get a Compromise Agreement, it would guarantee me a reference, and that is all I want out of it. I want to be gone, I want never to see her again, and I need a reference. It felt like a battle that I hadn't got myself into and yet I couldn't win, and that's the thing I hate most about it, the futility of it. You know, most people don't cause it, but they can't win, there's no way to win.

Emma recently told us: I have had an eventful year to say the least, but it's still been good as far as I'm concerned. The company

I was working for when I met you (teaching teenagers functional skills) went into liquidation in July and I was made redundant, but luckily through a contact I got another job within two weeks, still as a functional skills tutor, but working with unemployed adults this time. I really enjoyed that job, but unfortunately it also went into liquidation in November – I was very calm about it all this time, in part because I'd been there before and knew the process. I've had lots of support and friendship throughout, which is why I think it's been a good year, not a bad one!

I got a new job within a few days and am now a co-ordinator for functional skills, guiding a team of assessors on implementing the qualification within apprenticeships. It's like having a whole new career and has really got me enthused all over again! I do believe that, strangely enough, my experience with bullying actually made me a much stronger and ultimately happier, person – once I was able to deal with the issues that arose. I did need therapy, 6 months time off and some anti-depressants, so it wasn't all sunshine and roses, but the outcome was, if not worth it exactly, then at least a positive one!

4.6

Maria's story: potent relationships

Maria was an experienced Secondary school teacher, who had been teaching for 10 years.

Whenever I think back to my first teaching post at Colforth High School I remember what happened to Maria. It was just before Christmas, the kids were in a state of high excitement because end of term was near and it was snowing! I'd gone to ask her about the next lesson but I'd not been able to find her in the teaching rooms or the staffroom. I finally found her in the ladies toilets, sobbing her heart out.

'Maria! What's the matter?' She was unable to speak for a minute or two; she mopped her eyes, blew her nose and tried to regain her composure. 'I can't cope with it all any more', she wept. I wanted to comfort her but didn't like to put my arm around her; after all, although I was a mature entrant I hadn't been teaching very long, and she was very experienced and second in the department. 'What's it all about?' I asked.

'I can't do my job like this. David won't speak to me at all; he ignores me when he sees me. He sends me written instructions but won't let me ask him about them. He comes into my classroom, speaks to the kids and ignores me in front of them. Today he told me that there isn't enough Food Technology teaching to go round now and so I could either take a cut in my hours or I could teach PSHE[11]. So I said 'What is going to happen with Sandra, is she

_____

11   Personal, Social and Health Education

going to lose her hours as well?' He said, 'No.' I said I wasn't happy with that. If there was a shortage in hours then the unqualified staff should be the ones to lose hours first or to teach PSHE. He said, 'Well she can't teach PSHE because she's not qualified.' So I said, 'Well she's not qualified to teach Food Technology either, so how does that work?' She broke off at this point, too overcome by tears to speak.

Although it was only my second year I knew all the gossip about David and Sandra, what was going on outside school, and why he favoured Sandra, but I was still shocked to hear this latest news. David had been at the school for years, only becoming Head of Technology last year. He had seemed OK at first, a bit distant perhaps, but OK. Things were business-like although the atmosphere had seemed a little chilly. And then there were other things I'd heard: two years ago, Sandra, the sister-in-law of the previous HOD, came to work in the department as a technician. She had been interviewed for the job and all had seemed to be above board, but we didn't get much technical support from her. I think she just didn't really want to be a technician. She refused to do many of the jobs she was supposed to do. She was useless really! I knew that Maria had asked David, more than once, to ask her to do her jobs but he didn't support us: Maria started to get the silent treatment from both David and Sandra. And then last Christmas David announced that Sandra wanted to train as a teacher, and so she would be observing some lessons. Well, that was OK, I suppose, but I had thought it odd that she only ever observed Maria's classes. Then, last term, it got worse; David took 5 of Maria's lessons away and put her in as support in 5 of his GCSE lessons so that Sandra could 'try teaching'. I heard Maria say to David, 'Wouldn't it be better if Sandra was in the support role and I kept my teaching, because she hasn't been trained. It would be better for her, as well, in preparation for training as a teacher.' But David said, 'No.' He wanted her to try teaching.

I tried to give Maria some encouragement; 'Come on; don't

let it get you down. You're a brilliant teacher, the kids love you and you've got lots of good friends and support in the school. You mustn't give up. Perhaps you should talk to the Head.' She sighed deeply and then, with a catch in her voice, she said, 'I asked to see her at lunch time today but she was busy and she came to talk to me later while I was teaching a Y7 class, so I couldn't really talk about it properly. I said that I didn't think it was right to keep an unqualified teacher instead of a qualified one. The Head said 'that's just your opinion.' I told her I was going to speak to the Union again because I wasn't happy about this latest development. She was clearly not best pleased and accused me of going behind her back to the Union. Then she just walked off. They can do what they want – they are in the power position.'

I didn't know what to say. This all sounded very wrong. 'Perhaps you should speak to someone else about it,' I suggested. She said, 'Who else can I go to?'

I couldn't think of an answer so said, 'Look, it will be the end of term soon. Then you can have a good rest, get things into perspective. When you come back after Christmas things will look a lot better.'

Maria said, 'No, this is the final straw. I can't carry on any longer like this. I'm going.' She rushed blindly out of the toilets. I followed and watched as she picked up her bag and walked out of the building through the snow. She never came back.

I saw her in Tesco's about six months later. She seemed quite pleased to see me, and we had a bit of a chat. She told me that she had never understood why David fought so strongly for just one member of his department. She said, 'Other people who knew him well gave the obvious reason, and a previous Head of Department, who I have kept in touch with, said she thought he was having an affair with Sandra. I didn't really like to think it – but I guess that, looking back, they were probably right. It was a big risk for him to take, to favour an unqualified person over his highest performing department member.'

I still didn't understand why the Head supported him in getting rid of Maria and not Sandra. 'Well, it's cheaper to employ someone who they think will do just as good a job,' said Maria. I was shocked, 'Surely it's not just about cost?'

Maria sighed and said, 'It still fills me with distress that a teacher who never had any problems with pupils over a twelve year period, and was getting consistent pupil grades which were above their targets, and better year on year, was bullied out for the sake of a cheap, unqualified and unenthusiastic technician who wanted to teach and so was allowed to without relevant training or qualifications. I will never ever think that situation was an acceptable one under any circumstances, but the bottom line is that my health is more important than money.'

Maria recently told us: Sandra, the technician, is no longer teaching at the school and has returned to her role in technical support. There was not enough teaching for her because David's other friend, who had replaced Maria when she resigned, wanted to work full time. Sandra was good at sewing and upholstery but that wasn't what she was teaching. Maria could have understood it more if they'd put Sandra in technology doing textiles.

4.7

Andy's story: nothing's been the same since she came

Andy was 51, a well respected teacher, highly commended by Ofsted, who had been teaching at the same Primary school for 17 years. He was on the Senior Management Team (SMT), loved his job, and had good relationships with the children, the parents and the other members of staff. Two years after the arrival of a new Headteacher Andy had a complete mental breakdown and later took early retirement. During those two years there was an escalation of confrontations with, and accusations from, the Headteacher. The story begins a year after the new Headteacher arrived.

Why was it so quiet? Outside I could hear children playing but in here the big old clock ticked, and the tap in the kitchen corner dripped. I tried to eat my sandwiches silently. There was Andy, Deputy Head, at the table, head down as usual; Sally was pouring boiling water onto her Cuppa-Soup. Joan, the supply teacher was sitting next to me at the table. No-one was speaking. After a few minutes Sally broke the silence: 'I'm making tea, who wants a cup?' 'Yes please', chimed Andy, and the supply teacher.

The door opened, we all glanced up quickly, and then just as quickly looked away as Jane, the NQT, came in. The door closed behind her, shutting out the clatter of cutlery and the chatter of children from the hall opposite. No-one spoke. Jane pushed her long hair behind her ears as she took a large cardboard box out of her bag. One of her chewed finger nails was bleeding and her face was very pale. After some lengthy rustling, a plate with at least 12 pastries was set down on the table: 'Help yourselves, it's my birthday treat!' She attempted a smile but it couldn't hide the fact that she'd been crying again.

'Happy birthday, Jane! This is just what we need to keep us going,' Andy said, reaching for a cake. 'Come on everyone, cheer up. Let's wish Jane a happy birthday.' Sally took a cake and gave Jane a little smile. I took a pastry too, 'Thanks Jane.' Jane offered the plate to the supply teacher. 'You're new, aren't you? Have a cake'. The supply teacher took one, 'Oooh yummy! Thanks'. She looked at the plate and the remaining cakes. 'My word, you're generous aren't you – so many cakes!'

Jane bit her lip, looking towards the door before answering. 'Not really, there are a lot more staff but most people don't come in here at lunchtime. They'll pop in and get theirs later.' The supply teacher raised her eyebrows in surprise. 'Well, where I worked last term everybody was always in at lunchtime! It was a chance to relax and catch up on the gossip.' She turned to me, 'Is it always like this?'

'I couldn't say. I only started this year,' I said, but I knew the atmosphere was terrible. Everyone was walking on eggshells. By the end of last term people were hardly going into the staffroom. There was no Happy Christmas jollity. Everyone was very, very wary of saying anything because you could be overheard: the Head's room was next door. People always seemed on edge – quite different from my previous school. People here were always looking over their shoulder.

Jane sat looking at the cakes but didn't take one. 'Come on Jane, surely you've got room for one of your own birthday cakes,' Sally said. 'I don't think I can eat anything. I'm so worried about Monday, and I'm exhausted after all her learning walks; she's been in every day this week', Jane said, glancing again at the staffroom door. 'It's OK, Jane. She won't be coming in, she's got a parent with her at the moment.' said Sally.

'My class have been really hard work this week, and she's coming to observe me again on Monday.' Jane was looking tearful now. 'Don't worry, I'm sure things will get better when she's really settled in and got to know us', Andy advised, in his usual calm and steady way. 'It's all very well saying don't worry', said Sally, 'but we all know what she's doing to Jane – all those observations, constantly criticising her and telling her off, nothing's been the same since she came.'

'You know that questionnaire she sent round asking for views?' said Andy, 'Well, I handed mine in yesterday and I put that we desperately need to work on the morale of the staff in the school. She won't like it but at least she'll know that there's a problem and then I can talk to her about it.' Sally stared at him in amazement, pushing her hands through her tightly permed hair, 'Andy! I don't know how you dared! Nobody else has sent it back.'

'And don't forget what happened at the last staff meeting – and afterwards,' added Jane. 'We could hear her shouting at you through the wall; her office is next door.'

The supply teacher looked very interested, and asked, 'Why, what happened?'

'Well, you know, I've been at the school for a long time. I've always got on well with everybody here. I've never had a problem, and the parents are great. But since she came they've been asking what's going on. They can't get in to see her because she's put electric gates on the front of the school and moved her office right into the middle. You know, there are two doors you have to go through to get in? She won't talk to the parents and they are worried.'

'Because Andy's senior we asked him to speak about it in the staff meeting,' said Jane, 'and on top of that we wanted to know what she'd been telling the Governors about some of the things she'd been doing, and to get better communication going. So we'd already asked Andy to raise those questions.'

'Oh it was awful,' Sally whispered.

'Anyway,' said Andy, 'in the staff meeting I said I'd had a word with the rest of the staff and that none of us were happy about what the parents were saying, or about not getting any information from the Governors' meetings. She glared at me and said angrily 'Does anybody else agree with that?' The staff were terrified. Nobody said anything. She told us in no uncertain terms, that her policies and methods were staying just as they were, full stop. So I said, 'Well OK, but we are going to get trouble from the parents on some of this stuff'. Then everyone just looked at the floor – nobody said anything! And she stalked out.'

'I thought, Well, I'm on the management so I'd better go and talk to her. I went in and asked her if she would reassure the staff and parents. Then she started to rage at me and yelled: 'There's nothing wrong in this school!' I said, 'But there is Miss, you don't live in this town, I do. I am in contact through the rugby, the football, and all the other teams, and I know parents are concerned. The staff are too! And so are the children – it's affecting them too.'

She screamed at me, 'Oh get back to your class and close the door!', so I said OK, but there'll be trouble if you don't do something, and then I went back to my class.'

Just as Andy finished explaining, Mrs Harris, the Head, erupted into the room, leaving the door ajar. Children's shouts and laughter drifted into the silent staffroom. She sniffed the air. 'What can I smell? Oh, cakes! I've told you before not to bring cakes in here. They leave crumbs for mice.' She glanced around the table.

'Who brought those cakes in?' Jane's hands moved in the direction of the paper bag. 'Jane! I might have known! Those mice started in your room – I'm sure they were attracted by the food you kept in your cupboard. We've got mice everywhere in school now because of you and your cakes and biscuits.'

'I'm sorry Mrs Harris,' said Jane, gathering up the remains of pastries and taking them over to the bin.

'No! Not in there – take them out to the playground bins.' Jane stood still. Her hands shook and the bag rustled.

'Andy, I want to see you in my office now.' Jane was still

standing by the sink with the paper bag in her hand. 'Jane. Get rid of those cakes. Now!' said Mrs Harris. Jane turned and left the room. Everyone concentrated on the pattern of the carpet. Only the supply teacher continued eating her cake. No-one said a word as Andy got up and followed Mrs Harris out of the room. Then the shouting began.

We heard the door slam when Andy eventually marched out. He never came back.

Andy recently told us: I've heard that a male NQT has felt the full force of her obsession with getting her own way. She's hounded him each day, resulting in him breaking down in tears in front of other members of staff and eventually, two or three weeks ago, actually walking out of the school.

Andy still finds himself looking back as if it was yesterday, and feels that a part of him has died. When he 'finished' he never even got a wave goodbye! He believes that the Headteacher abused her position, which will always leave a bad taste in his mouth, hanging over him forever, knocking his confidence in every walk of his life. However, his ambition is to eventually shake off the constant drudgery of depression, and he consoles himself by believing that somehow fate will deliver appropriate judgement upon his Headteacher, and that maybe she will see how she has destroyed people's lives – some sort of retribution!

5

THE SENIOR
MANAGERS'
RESPONSES

A Primary Head Teacher's reaction to Emma's account

The scenario you've given me is of a consistently good or better teacher, with 15 years of experience, who actually wants to stay in teaching rather than progress to become a Deputy or a Head. So, she sounds from that as if she'd be the sort of teacher anybody would want to employ.

The morale in the school is low and it seems that the reason for the morale being low is the Head. This is a very familiar scenario to me. I have worked in a school where teachers cried in the stock cupboards. This teacher is very quickly being demoralised and deskilled. You've got a teacher who's gone into the school, a very experienced and very good teacher, and it's taken no time at all to knock the confidence out of her. And she wouldn't be performing to the best of her ability, not how she would normally perform. So the Head goes in, and does an observation of a teacher who isn't actually doing what she would normally do. This teacher needed to be given breathing space.

Being told off in front of the staff, that is very unprofessional behaviour. If the Head had something to say to a member of staff then she should say, 'Oh, can you pop into my room, there's something I'd like to have a chat with you about.' It almost sounds as if it's the Head who's on the brink of a nervous breakdown herself, because she's demoralised the staff. The staff are frightened to say anything to her.

You've got some bad practice here, because the verbal feedback on her performance, at a performance management meeting, was that she'd met all her targets, and nothing else was said. What she should have received was a written report shortly after, and it should have reflected what was said verbally. So there shouldn't have been a mismatch, and the written report should have come at the same time or very shortly afterwards. There's a culture of fear in this school isn't there? At least Emma summoned up the courage to ask the Head directly if she had any issues, which was good, and it must have taken some courage on her part to be able to do that.

The Head's trying to manipulate the situation by getting her to leave, rather than going through formal procedures. I can understand that lots of Heads would do that, because going through formal procedures is a lengthy, difficult process. But it's not very professional.

I don't think she was right to suggest Capability Procedures. It sounds to me as if she took on a very good teacher and managed to demoralise her to such an extent that she may well have became a less good teacher, but only because of the way she was treated.

Accepting a Compromise Agreement is a good escape route for Emma. She could leave the school and not lose her good reputation, but it allows the Head to carry on being a bully. So, it's addressing Emma's needs, but it's not addressing the bigger picture. I think a lot of Heads get away with things, again and again and again, because that happens.

This scenario has many elements similar to something that I experienced first-hand. I could have become bullied had I not been stronger. I was certainly demoralised, very quickly. I had taught in a couple of schools in challenging areas with really challenging children, but in those schools the staff were really well supported.

And then I got a job in a leafy, middle-class type school, and I hadn't heard about the reputation of this Head, but apparently it was out there in the world. When I mentioned to a couple of colleagues, 'Oh, I'm starting at so and so school in September.' There was a sharp intake of breath, and they said, 'Well, we've heard rumours about the Head there.' I was bright and breezy and said, 'Ok I'll take her as I find her,' because she had seemed very nice when I went and visited. So I started at the school, and I very quickly learned through the rumour mill that a member of staff had taken her to the Union, in a very similar scenario to Emma's. The Head had paid the member of staff off, and written her a good reference, but the school had a huge staff turnover, which always rings alarm bells. Every week there would be a member of staff crying in the stock cupboard, or sobbing in the corner of the staffroom, and it was mainly because the Head really wanted every member of staff to be a clone of herself and didn't allow for any individuality, or creativity. Everything had to be done the way she would do it, if she were that teacher. And obviously I came under criticism, just the same as everybody else did. I wasn't singled out, because everybody was treated as badly. I suppose the difference was that I would on occasion go to her and would say can we talk about what I was unhappy about, but she didn't respond well, because I don't think she was used to having a professional challenge.

Although I was being fairly thick-skinned about it, it was getting me down, so by the October half-term I thought, no, I can't stay here, this isn't the school for me. I'd only been there a couple of months. By the last day of May I hadn't got a job to go to, but I handed in my notice anyway, because I just thought if I stay in this school it will make me ill, and so I moved on.

So, not unlike Emma's situation, I went into this school as a highly regarded, very able teacher, which is why she'd employed me, and straight away so many things that I was doing were in her eyes wrong. It wasn't targeted just at me, because other teachers were in the same boat. There was a real climate of fear in the school, with people looking over their shoulders. And people wouldn't do anything because they would try to second guess how would this Head react, if I said this, if I did this, or if I put this display up like this. So yes, I have every sympathy with Emma.

5.2

A Primary Head Teacher shares her experiences of dealing with bullies

Yes, I've certainly experienced this sort of thing. Somebody that I knew from student days came to my school as a Head and I became her Deputy, and it was in this role as Deputy that the bullying started. I endured all sorts of unpleasant situations like overhearing her talking about me, because I'd had a cold, and it was, 'Oh, poor her!' Just unpleasant playground type behaviour, talking about me to other people. I think she was jealous because I had such a high standing in the school and I had been there for so long, and the parents loved me, and the staff loved me, as you do when you've worked with people for a long time. And they didn't have that feeling for her and I think it was sort of, 'They like you better than me, so I'm not going to be nice to you.' It was that type of behaviour.

I got breast cancer, so I had to have time off, and she kept phoning me up and saying, 'I need to know when you're coming back.' I was obviously not in a very good place at the time, and I was going to chemotherapy, and she kept insinuating that I wouldn't have a job to go back to, and then all of a sudden I got this letter from Occupational Health and they just seemed to be under the impression that I wasn't fit for work. I felt that somebody had been telling them that I wasn't fit for work rather than having an open conversation to see how well I was. And when I did go back to speak to her at the school, she effectively told me that I wouldn't go back to my own class, the class that I'd had, she was going to allow the supply teacher to stay and that I would be a floating person and I would have two days here and there, and the job that she was offering me was appalling. I was the Deputy, so I turned the tables on her, I was so angry, and I don't normally get angry, I can't bear confrontation, but I spoke through anger and I said, 'you have got your priorities completely wrong as Head of this school. I should be the person that you are nurturing and thinking about being loyal to, not a supply teacher, and I am going to have my class back because if I don't, you can be sure that this story is going to be publicised, I don't care who I have to go to but your actions here in this room are going to be known. And she backtracked totally and I got my class back, but she was a bit wary of me after that.

That Head had a way of manipulating people so that you actually didn't know about it until you spoke to somebody else. I became very friendly with another leading teacher at the school and the Head didn't like that, and she did her utmost to break us up. I mean it was just all really petty stuff. She told this other teacher that I had done or said things, and that I wanted her to do this particular task that she was handing out, and when we actually got to chatting it wasn't like that at all, I'd said something else, and in the end we were comparing notes about what was being said to us in confidence in the office and we realised what was going on, and it was a real sort of planned divide and rule. I don't know what her aim was, other than to try and make herself look good in the school. No-one complained she was a bully!

But she was acting like a bully, doing these things, always in her room with the door closed, and there was just you and her, and you'd come out and think, 'Did that just happen?' I suppose she assumed that we wouldn't talk about it to each other but we did, although it was a while before we did! We put up with lots of things separately, not realising that this was going on. It's horrible talking about it actually because it brings back the feelings of it. She stayed with us for about 5 years then got a job in another school.

I took over as Head. But she left behind terrible, terrible things that we discovered when we looked in her accounts. Financially, we found a huge deficit that we knew nothing about. So I think possibly she felt she was losing it in the school.

But this sort of story is quite common. It is sad, and it's so commonplace, honestly, the people that have spoken to me about it. It can happen at any level. A friend of mine, who's not teaching now, was a Head at the same time as I was (we met on the same NPQH course) and she was bullied out by her Governors. She had a mental breakdown and hasn't worked since.

I once had a student who was being bullied by one of my teachers, a teacher that you would never have thought – well, actually I have an inkling that she was a bit power crazy, and she's a Head now. When she was in my school she was sweetness and light with everybody, but this student just kept breaking down in tears, and one day I was told by one of the TAs, who came running in to me as the Head, saying that this girl was in the cupboard crying. So I went into the cupboard and got her out saying, 'I just need to have a word with you in my office about something.' So I took her and I asked, 'What on earth's happening?', and I found out that the teacher had been bullying her and saying she would never make a teacher. Effectively she was being told that she was rubbish, and every day she was having this said to her, and still trying to perform with the children, but I had no idea it was going on. So, I had the teacher in, and I said, 'You are the only person who's seeing this side of this student. I've watched her work with the children, and the TAs, and all the adults that are involved with her have said, 'Yes. She's not there yet, but she's got a lovely manner with the children, she's prepared for the lesson that she's doing and she talks to them, she interacts and she's trying to push them along in their learning'. They've all had good things to say, so where are you coming from with your 'She's never going to…'? Did you actually say to her she's never going to succeed?' The teacher said, 'Oh well I may have said it in a fit of pique or something,' and I said, 'You can't do that with human beings. You've actually driven that girl into the cupboard crying, what does that say about you as a human being? Where's that coming from?' And she said, 'Oh I was having a really bad day, I didn't realise she had taken it to heart.'

I told her that if you are in charge of a nursery and reception class combined, you are also in charge of a lot of adults, and you can't treat people like that. That if she can't treat people in a better way then she'd have to come out of the job and go into one of the other classrooms, because I can't have her as a manager of staff if she can't communicate with people in a more positive way. If she had issues with the student, to that extent, then she should have come and spoken to me about it and we'd have tried to do something together, because that student needs support. She said, 'Oh, I'm sorry, I'm sorry, I didn't realise it had affected her. Perhaps we'd better all get together then.' So we did. I got the student in, and the teacher concerned actually ended up crying, saying she was so sorry, and didn't realise what she'd said, and after that it seemed to be OK. I think she just got above herself; the being in charge of people was having an adverse effect on her personality. And the student passed her teaching practice!

Two Secondary school Managers talk about Jo's story

Manager 1

Lots of people refer to things like what happened to Jo and Erica as personality clashes. That's the difficulty. And what you haven't got is Erica's version of what happened. Erica could well have been put into a HOD position, unable to manage Jo, and perhaps she hadn't been given management skills to manage Jo, so she fell back on isolating her, basically, and managing it very, very badly.

Apart from anything else, Erica is totally unprofessional and should be held to account for her actions. Jo's gone to Pam, who's the Deputy, and made a complaint, but nothing's changed. So Pam obviously wasn't terribly effective. It's good that she made a formal complaint. The difficulty is that there is no account as to why Erica has done these things. And even if she has done them for good reasons, she can't manage Jo, she's been unprofessional in the way that she's done things, and that shouldn't happen. It looks as though Erica went to another school. So presumably she was fobbed off somewhere else. That's not terribly uncommon, that story.

One of the problems is that people like Heather her line manager, and Pam the Deputy Head, at that stage in their career, quite often they've gone through some basic management training, but they probably haven't touched upon how to deal with very difficult things like bullying in the workplace, grievance procedures, and all those things. And lots of staff are in Deputy Headships and assistant Headships and HODs and they've got no training in that whatsoever. The availability of training depends very much on your LA, and it differs from LA to LA, and it also depends on whether you perceive training as something that you ought to go on, as a Head and Deputy. Quite often it's down to your perception of what you need to go and get trained in. So you are likely to go and get the Ofsted training, the framework, you're likely to go and get assessment and data. But do you actively seek some of these things out? It may be that you might do them as a kneejerk reaction to something that happens. Competing against targets and being driven for children to achieve tends to be the focus, and consequently personnel issues are not always high on the list, although safeguarding would be very high because that's part of the Ofsted criteria.

Personnel issues are very difficult to deal with and there are some people who are in management positions who either haven't been trained, or they haven't got their own personal set of skills to be able to deal with these things, or they find it quite intimidating. Maybe that Deputy Head didn't have the inclination to go and tackle Erica (HOD) even though she shouldn't have acted in that way as it was totally unprofessional. There is one thing, when Jo came to look at the student's lesson plan and they'd changed it, and then she had to continue teaching, when Erica said, 'Oh yes, we changed it,' but without telling her, that's wrong, but it happens every day because life changes so quickly in school. Jo would have seen that as totally undermining, and probably would have felt that her HOD didn't care about her, and therefore didn't bother to tell her. It may not have been that, but regardless, the set of skills that the HOD showed were poor.

What Jo's story shows is that some managers don't have the ability to manage difficult situations. It could be a lack of people skills, or it could be because they don't have policies and procedures in place. And it could also be something that is experienced more *and more, that the demands on the managers are so great that they become dismissive when they deal with other people. That's not to say it's right, but it happens, and 10 years ago you saw it mostly in Secondary schools when there was such a big thrust to move failing Secondary schools onwards, and there was Ofsted notice to improve. When that happened, the demands on Managers to shift things on were so great that they themselves became harder, and perhaps put time and people skills aside because they're target driven. It's far worse now, it's moved further into Primary schools. And it happens more with bigger organisations because you have a distanced management structure.*

Manager 2

It's a failure in process isn't it? It was very ineffective. You don't know whether the Head had Erica in to talk about this, but it seems that this is unprofessional isn't it, no doubt about it. If you look in the Teacher Standards and if you look in the old GTCE standards there is reference to generic things that a teacher expects in relation to their colleagues, and that sort of thing is just overlooked here. I think Jo did the right thing in noting all the things down, because if a member of staff came to a Senior Manager and said she thought she was being bullied by someone they would ask, 'What evidence have you got?' And if they hadn't got any evidence they would say, 'Right, Ok. It's not that I don't believe you, but if you want me to confront somebody I need to confront them with something. So either keep a note of what's going on and then bring it to me as soon as something happens again, or you go home and you think about what it is and you identify all those things and I'll tackle it first thing tomorrow morning, because I'm not going to let it go any further.' So, Jo did the right thing in doing that, but she hasn't got enough support throughout, either from Heather, or Pam. And the fact that Erica left so suddenly, probably the Head gave her a compromise reference.

It's a really interesting thing and it does seem to be bullying. There's been a system failure that hasn't effectively, at lower levels, nipped in the bud something which should have been dealt with at a very low level. And if members of staff are being publicly denigrated by other members of staff, in front of staff or in front of children, that's unacceptable, and straight away that would be it. There would be questions: 'Right, this has happened – has this happened? Witness statements?', to see if that was the case, and if that was the case then, 'Right, first of all I'm giving you an informal warning that this has happened. If it happens again then it will become a formal, oral warning.' There's a discipline process to go to, to do with these matters. Erica should have been disciplined.

Some Heads may not be properly prepared for the role they're taking on. In pre-academy days, the LA offered a package of sessions as induction for a Head. A part of that was the grievance procedure, disciplinary matters, meeting the Unions, talking to the Unions, and so there was a pretty good induction. And, in addition to that, every new Head was assigned a kind of coach or a mentor, so that they could talk to someone who was an experienced Head from outside their area. There are briefings that the Secondary Heads of the LA do, even now. They have a half-termly Secondary Heads Conference and a Primary Heads Conference, at which key issues are brought up. But it's the attitude of the Head towards these matters. If the Head wants an easy life in the first instance, it's easy to sweep these things under the carpet, but if you want to have a school where people feel valued, and people feel recognised and people are happy to come to school, and do a good job for you, you have to tackle these matters head on and be professional about it. And the middle leaders need help to understand that if they are to be professionals in the profession, they have to act professionally with their staff, because they deserve it. Sometimes we don't get it right. I'm the first to say there are some times when I get it wrong, but it's always a learning experience.

5.4

Two Primary school Managers talk about Jenny, Emma, and the problem of references

Manager 1

Clearly 8.25 in the morning is not the best time to go in and discipline a teacher, as if you could just teach children for the rest of the day while now feeling inadequate and upset! You can say to someone, 'Oh, can I have a word with you?' and they might become really worried and upset, so Heads learn not to say that, or to say, 'I need to talk to you about such and such,' because it's a realisation that what you say affects people in a way that perhaps it hasn't before. Maybe that's something that a new Head needs to understand. And it's likely that there would be issues with behaviour management, in a class like that, for any teacher, but particularly a young and relatively inexperienced teacher like Jenny, to have that mix, and autism with ADHD. These are really specific things that you would want people to have had training for, to have read books, to have had team teacher training – all of those sorts of things. There was certainly a lack of skill in management, maybe the ability wasn't there, or the Head actually needs training, or is just a bully. It's certainly bullying type behaviour.

Obviously the Head wasn't very pleased with what she saw, but if alarm bells had rung in her head then maybe she should have put some support in place. There's absolutely no excuse for going into the room at 8.25 in the morning to talk to Jenny. What she should have done is to have said, 'Can we get together at such and such a time to chat about…', but not as this poor girl is about to start her working day.

As a Head, if you are going to have that difficult conversation, you've got to have very smart targets, such as, 'This is what I've observed, and this is what we could do to put it right; perhaps some training towards that, but at the end of the day this is what I want next time I observe you, and to see how you're doing it differently.' But neither Jenny nor Emma were given any specific targets to work on, so again, that's not good practice. At the end of the day if staff are not getting something right the best way to help them is to support them, not to criticise them. New Heads, like any other new person, are learning on the job, especially if they are brand new to post and haven't been a Head before. But it sounds as if this new Head is actually quite stressed herself and doesn't actually know how to deal with staff, doesn't know how to support staff.

Jenny and Emma clearly became more and more demoralised, which probably had a knock-on effect on their behaviour, so they were unlikely to be managing their classes as they might have done if they hadn't continually had the Head looking over their shoulders, and likely as not criticising.

It sounds as if the Head was setting Jenny up to fail when she was given this peripatetic role, to cover other teachers and classes, because most wouldn't give that sort of a role to someone who was in their early years of teaching. The Head here is giving out inconsistent messages because, despite earlier criticisms, in early October she observed a music lesson and gave Jenny feedback that her behaviour management had improved. And yet, when she had the performance management meeting, less than a month later, it was still deemed in need of improvement. The Head raised the threat that Jenny could go into Capability, so the first thing that she should do is contact her Union representative, because really she is being treated quite badly. On the one hand, morally the right thing to do would be to challenge the Head for bullying, but being pragmatic you don't shoot yourself in the foot and possibly jeopardise your future job. So the kindest thing that you could say about the Head was that she wasn't really doing her job properly. But, in reality, I think that the Head not doing her job properly was resulting in her being a bully, and that she really badly managed this teacher.

Manager 2

There is a catalogue of things in Jenny's story about the leaving party, completely unacceptable behaviour. Everything appears to have been going fine for her until the new Head arrived (and it was the same for Debbie, despite her history of clinical depression). It really is very sad. There are, unfortunately, too many Heads that do this sort of thing. I know of at least 3 who do it on purpose. The first thing they decide is to get rid of the old staff because they want their own ones in, ones they can mould to the way they want the school to be, so they can make their mark. And it is easily done in a school, because you haven't got a massive big place of work where they can go somewhere else. And this poor girl, frightened to do anything, because where do you go for your reference? You have to get one from your last Head.

I know of a teacher who hasn't worked for many years, because the reference she was given by her Head has been following her around. She can't get a job because they keep going on that last reference. She's taken courses, done supply where she can but she still hasn't worked properly. Her previous Head effectively destroyed her life. She did try to get a copy of the Head's reference but she wasn't allowed access to it. And here's another example, when I needed a reception class teacher. The panel had a phenomenally good interview with one girl but we got a terrible reference from her last school, plus I got a phone call from her Head who said, 'I couldn't put it all on your reference form but I felt you ought to know...' And then the vitriol that came out of her mouth about this girl! It's not a healthy situation. Although I would have gone with this girl the others on the interview panel wouldn't, and this poor girl is still trying to get a job, and she is really, really good at her job, but this one person is successfully preventing her from doing it, that is evil isn't it? At least Jenny escaped that fate.

5.5

Senior Managers' combined talk about strong personalities and power

Several teachers' accounts were read by a number of Senior Managers, all of whom made some points in common. In this account their comments have been combined into one coherent narrative.

Well, I know how Andy feels, being the only one to speak out. His new Head is the kind of person I worked for, for 2 years. I had someone punch my desk and shout, 'What the f****ing hell am I going to do with you,' and I'd been threatened. I could have gone away and cried, because I'm not very strong, but in the end I changed my job, because that was the easiest thing to do; of course it would be harder for Andy – I was a lot younger than he is. Eventually my Head was suspended for bullying, and for shouting and swearing at the teachers.

Could it be because of Andy's strong personality? He was on the SMT, everybody knew him. If he was very popular, and people were coming and telling him things then perhaps she thought, 'They should be telling me that!' There's no kind of leadership by example here, is there? It's all very authoritarian, and no attempt at other leadership styles to get people on board, to win over hearts and minds.

The whole thing about power, about perceived power as opposed to actual power, is interesting: you could have a strong personality, perhaps, in a member of staff who, because they've

*got the strength of personality, if they disagree, or they don't like
something, they could make life quite difficult for somebody senior
to them. There are some people who don't realise how influential
they are, and there's something about them, that they are able to
influence the opinions and actions of others. And it's important
for the Head, for the senior leadership to be aware of who those
people are, because that needs to be channelled. If it is channelled
properly it can be a really useful tool for the school. But I know
that, in the past, I've had to take people to one side and say, 'Do
you know that when you talk about some of these things you
can bring the whole atmosphere of the whole school down, and
actually you could be a real positive force for good in the school.'
I'm thinking of a specific time where that person went away and
thought about it, and then came back and wanted to talk more,
and I was able to explain, 'Well, you know, it's not that I want to
stop you,' because the initial thing was that he believed that I was
stopping him saying things, having an opinion. I said, 'No, I don't
want to stop you having an opinion, but maybe you've got strong
opinions, and when something happens you've got an opinion
about, perhaps you could come and talk to me and we can see if
there's a way round it,' and I asked for reasoning and things like
that, before he stirred the whole hornets' nest up.*

*However, people who have lost perspective on life shouldn't be
Heads. If they've worked their way up to that, and they've managed
to go through all those channels, then at that point maybe control
is everything, and this person does have control issues. Then if you
don't do as they say they can't cope with it. You know, you're going
to get as many ill and sick Heads as you are other people in the
other professions.*

*The questionnaire was supposed to be anonymous, parents
were complaining, and electric gates? For heaven's sake! And all
those other incidents he's told you about – trying to enforce total
silence on children at dinner time, her throwing his things on the
floor and shouting at him in front of the children and staff, that*

really is totally unprofessional – poor chap. There is a really serious problem with the Head here, her staff are terrified and no-one will say anything. What is scary is that Andy has taken it on but the other staff haven't, they are still there suffering, complaining, but not doing anything about it.

Appeals and grievances are very difficult, very hard. If a school has been moved on in terms of attainment and Ofsted success, then Heads or school Governors might justify their actions for such results. Andy could go to the Union, take out a grievance (which I see he did a year into his sickness absence), but by leaving, like I did, teachers mostly have 'given in'. Taking out a grievance, which is heard by the Governors, is always a really nasty thing to do, it's dreadful for the school but sometimes you just have to do it. Andy (and Maria) would need to have had all the evidence listed, dates and everything. Unfortunately, Andy lost his grievance, but at least the employment tribunal eventually found in his favour and he got the money he was owed that the Head was withholding, brilliant. In the end he takes early retirement, poor chap.

In Maria's case, well it's really about the way it was done. Being rude to her, humiliating her, the fact that her Head made her cry, you just don't do that. How does that make people improve? The apparent ongoing 'special relationship' between Maria's technician and her Head of Department shares similarities with my experiences as a young teacher, pre-Headship. I was bullied by my Head and I didn't know where to turn to either. In the end I complained to the Head of Primary Education in my LA, only to find out that that person was in a relationship with my Head, so I didn't get very far with it. I found it really difficult, and I nearly went under because I didn't really know who to turn to during that period, or what to do, but eventually the problem was solved because my husband and I moved house. But Maria was the breadwinner in the family; she couldn't escape by just leaving. As a fulltime qualified teacher she didn't understand why an unqualified teacher, her technician, should get paid to teach while she is given other work, not the subject she is qualified for.

There may be other difficult relationships in Maria's story, and we don't know how Sandra (the technician) felt or what she was doing throughout this. But it is being badly managed – appallingly managed – and the leadership of the department should have been criticised by Ofsted if they knew all this was happening. And where is the Head in all this? But Ofsted probably wouldn't be able to pick up on any of this, and Maria might have left by then anyway. It seems a very sad situation and it seems a muddle. Maria feels bullied, but you don't know the background to this. Andy's story seems more straightforward, while Maria's seems much more tangled. Maybe they just didn't want her at the school anymore. If there were really serious relationship problems then they may just have wanted to get rid of her, and offered a deal to make it happen.

5.6

Managers' combined talk about pressures, proper procedures, support and costs

It's possible that more staff perceive they are being bullied now, but I think that is as a result of the increasing demands for better and better results. There is also a changing Ofsted framework that means if your judgement goes down to 'satisfactory' the school could be in a tailspin. The impact could last three years, with the number of students going down, reduced resourcing and staff, and all of those things. Unfortunately the top-down pressure for higher performance, for more and more out of the staff, means that there is a very fine line, confusion even, between bullying and increasing demand.

I do think that the pressure on reaching targets and the changing Ofsted criteria, etc, has actually made Heads harder, much harder. You have to be hard and deliver those hard messages. But Heads of Department, Deputy Heads and Heads are not always skilled up to do so. There's a really fine balance between coaching and supportive leadership, and leadership where you say, 'These are my expectations and you have to live up to them.'

Ofsted doesn't tend to look at staff turnover at all, or at morale. They're focused on achievements, behaviour, parental opinion of the school, and they're focused on the spiritual, moral and cultural experience of the children. What they don't do is talk to the staff about what it's like to teach in this school.

But if you've got a difficulty then you've got policies and procedures that you could and should use, and you've got a set of personal management skills that you can use. You should use all of those in a supportive manner. If you don't, then ultimately no, you're not doing your job properly. But it's very, very tough doing it. Heads are subject to a huge amount of stress themselves, and I think one of the really difficult things, as I've now discovered, is not passing all that stress to your staff. Some Heads are better at it than others.

There is a way to approach a teacher in a professional and supportive way, and if the support is not working then that person has representation. If you play it by the book, which is what you should do, then you should have an informal meeting to tell them that you've got some concerns, and ask how you can support them. Then have a period of support to help that person, support which is genuine, where you don't undermine people. If there is still no improvement, then you start the formal procedures, and you say, 'Look, we still don't believe that you're making that improvement, we've still got concerns about X, Y and Z.' But that person should have been asked to have her Union representative or colleague to come in with them. The first meeting would be the beginning of informal capabilities, before they can go to Capability, with every bit of support that the teacher says they need to improve put in place. A teacher can bring their Union to any meeting with their Head, at any point, if they wish to. Usually it happens because you advise them to do it, and often that's the first hint that actually this is quite a serious issue, whatever the issue is.

Initially it would be a private conversation because there might well be barriers to the meeting and the fulfilling of targets. So, that conversation would take place, and be noted on the performance management form. I would expect my middle and senior leaders to take a note of it personally. They might back it up with an email, just to say, 'We've discussed this matter and this is what we covered.' But if, over the course of time, nothing is changing despite the strategy being put in place, then the question would become a bit more formal, 'OK. We're still not getting anywhere, what are *you going to do?' If my middle leader is saying to me, 'Actually, they're making no progress at all. The class is in danger of missing it's targets altogether – and we've had two meetings,' performance management would then be my responsibility. I would look at the notes of the meetings and say, 'OK then it's time to make it more formal. She can invite her Union official if she wants to. Let's talk about the issue, what's happened, what needs to be done, are we doing enough,' and give the opportunity to hear their side of the story, for me to get a fuller understanding, because I get things third party. It would be a formal conversation because as soon as it comes to me, generally, things become more formal.*

I know that I wouldn't see any improvement in the 4 weeks that Gove (former Secretary of State for Education) has suggested unless there was something very, very specific. It is probably legally right but I think it's too short term. Maybe 6 to 8 weeks or half a term is probably the right amount of time for a teacher to show progress, and you'd want them to make progress. The need to do proper performance management, or appraisal, or call it what you will, then becomes an imperative of that process. At the first sign of trouble, whether it's formal or informal, it has to be noted down, because the Unions will say, 'Well you haven't done it on performance management.'

After six weeks absence you'd generally send them to OH. You have to get the permission of the teacher for OH to write to their GP, who then sends stuff to OH. Then they interview them and a report is written to the Head, the school, and back to their GP. My experience has been, both personally and through Headship, that OH are very sympathetic. I have, as a Head, recommended and paid for counselling for some members of staff. I've got a limited budget, and 6 sessions is £300, but if you can get a member of staff back, then it's good. If you really think there is a grievance then it's got to be looked at. Often there is a counter-grievance, and the policy says that if there is a counter-grievance it will be investigated separately after the initial one. Sometimes a grievance is over a really petty matter, and they do run the risk that at the end there is no grievance, no case to answer. It is quite complicated, they have to be right in their own mind about what's happened because other people's reputations are at risk, and to believe just the story of one without a full investigation into the wider narrative is not to undertake your duty. The main thing is whether the person who's making the grievance believes it to be something that has actually happened and warrants investigation, because to take somebody off timetable for nearly 5 days is very expensive.

The idea that if you take formal proceedings you can no longer give a good reference isn't true either. If you were moving into Capability, even when you're into Capability, there's always the chance they can turn it round, so you can't ever say I'm not going to give you a good reference, it's not automatic. And if you go for a Compromise Agreement then you sit down and you agree together what the reference is going to say, so it can be quite a fair reference.

Local authorities definitely have a role to play in the induction of teachers because they see all the NQTs, and they should be making them very aware of the school's wellbeing helpline, which you can ring about anything that's bothering you. Every school has to buy into a wellbeing programme. We buy into the county one, it's not terribly good but it's reasonably inexpensive. My colleague buys into a much better one, but all of them will have a line that's about your wellbeing.

Support for Heads is very bitty, and is quite quickly withdrawn if they think you're coping. A good mentor can be fantastic, but of course you don't necessarily have a good mentor, and mentors are existing Heads who have their own huge workloads. But what happens is you go to a Heads' conference or some training, and after a while you get to know other Heads. Usually the best bit of support is the chit-chat that you have in the break, that little bit of networking. New Heads coming to the profession haven't yet joined that little informal group. If you're the sort of Head who doesn't have enough confidence to make those networking connections, or to pick up the phone and say, 'Look, I'm really struggling with dah de dah, what are you doing about it,' or 'Can we get together and have a chat about...', then you're keeping all that stress in, and perhaps you can fall into the trap of just loading all that stress onto your staff.

There's this irony, that they can't find enough Heads, that nobody wants the job, and yet nobody seems to have put together the fact that Heads aren't being supported and nurtured and looked after with the fact that nobody really wants the job. You are judged all the time, and under enormous pressure to provide. Parents expect more, the LA expects more, Ofsted expects more. Your staff expect an awful lot more than I ever expected from a Head 30 years ago, so the pressures are enormous. You're answerable to everybody but nobody is interested in you. I suspect it's that sense of pressure and accountability that filters down and spills over, and causes some of these situations to not be handled properly. Because if your Governors are nagging you about your GCSE results, or in my case your SATs results, and so is the LA, and you've got parents nagging you about something else, the fact that you apply unreasonable pressure to somebody below you, well, I can see that that would happen.

It's about change in accountability. It's only since Ofsted has come, as an outside agency that's going to come in and judge your school, and it doesn't matter what anybody says, it's the Head, at the end of the day, that takes most of the flak when it comes. If it's a good Ofsted it's the Head that's seen in lights, and if it's a bad Ofsted it's still down to the Head. Whatever you do you can't get away from that. If your school comes out badly they will remove you. So, because the pressure's so high on Heads it gets filtered down, and unfortunately that sometimes comes with the impression that you might be bullying somebody.

The Government needs to back off basically, they don't tell business men how to run businesses but they tell Heads how to run schools. By and large 90% of us do a bloody good job and we just want to be left to do it. We love the kids and I think we're paid fairly. I don't think for 1 minute I'm underpaid but I do work for every half penny. If only the Government would just leave us to get on with it! The competitive nature of the workplace is worse. We've now got an academy, a free school and a maintained high school servicing one area, so what used to be partnership working is now competitive. That goes into a kind of capitalist society and accountability and league tables, and if you're not top you're failing, but we aren't a product industry. So, to be perfectly honest, it is such a mess that I don't think there is any one thing that could happen that's going to change it, other than the Government saying, 'Right, for the next 5 years we won't change anything.'

6

THE UNION
COMMENTARIES

6.1

Union officials' confirmation of bullied teachers' experiences

Types of bullying

We've come across almost all of the things mentioned in these teachers' stories: a general atmosphere of nothing you can do is ever right, the unannounced observations, the grading as unsatisfactory. They're all things that come up every day. Recently a teacher was told off because she didn't have a pencil monitor in the class! It's really quite trivial stuff but it builds up. Yes, a lot of the teachers' stories are very familiar. Things like turning up unannounced for observations, implied criticism without any basis, or without anything explicit, all these sorts of things ring very true. And a feeling that although they've done nothing wrong, were not failing in any way, but being so undermined that actually, in the end, the only thing that they can think of doing is getting out.

It's the nature of the profession, when they're being dealt with inappropriately or in a bad way by their employer, that they don't tell anybody, they don't raise it, they carry on; they hope that if they keep their heads down, work harder and harder, then the bully, the harasser, the Head will move their target. Quite often what happens is that when it becomes intolerable and they have a complete breakdown, we go into the school looking for corroborative witness testimony and it's not there, even from their friends and people that they've worked with for a long time.

It's because they don't want to get involved, they still have to earn a wage and develop a career in that particular school. So, if we're unable to say to the Head: ' Look, we raised this issue with you, we raised the fact that you were dealing with that person inappropriately, that her workload was excessive, recorded the fact that we'd raised it,' and in effect put the employer on notice, then it's almost impossible, actually, to retrieve the position.

New heads

It's very common for teachers to phone up about bullying when there's a new Head. When Heads come into a new role, they want to stamp their own mark, to be seen to do things differently, and teachers being asked to do something differently doesn't mean they're being bullied. Sometimes it's a case of, 'Oh we've always done it like this,' but it's not necessarily unreasonable if you're being asked to change some things. We know that all new Heads make changes, and sometimes people perceive that as bullying. Sometimes it is bullying, but sometimes it's not. For example, we have cases where Heads have worked with somebody for twenty years, failed to deal with some issues, and the new Head comes in and deals with it, and that's not bullying.

Getting rid

With older, more expensive teachers a lot of Heads of schools out there are thinking: right, we've got to get our money's worth out of them, and you might find that there's a bit more pressure on them to achieve a bit more. They might find themselves subject to a few more observations, or there's a threat of Capability held over them, and yes, older teachers are a bit more vulnerable. It is really common to hear, 'I've never had any problems before, I've been a teacher for thirty years, I've always been good,' and then all of a sudden it's no, you're not. That in itself can completely undermine almost everything that they feel they've ever done and they're devastated, absolutely devastated.

We do see schools getting rid of teachers by using the Capability Procedure, because it's easy to do that. They're using it to get rid of older teachers because they're too expensive to keep, and they are getting in new, younger, cheaper ones that they think they can train and nurture along their own lines. But of course they haven't got that background, that experience and it's tragic actually, because you're losing that wealth of experience.

If a school has concerns about a teacher then they should assist them in the first place. But after that, if there were still issues to be addressed then, quite rightly, they should move into a formal process. But what you find is that they'll either seek to pursue it in a very aggressive way, undermining the confidence of teachers, or the teacher will go sick, long term, and then they'll be managed out of the system. We see loads of instances of that.

Controlling heads

It's very difficult to rebut a Head's concerns, because clearly if they've got concerns they should raise them with teachers. But when it's being done to bully and attack somebody it's very difficult to prove it's that, rather than a genuine concern. If a person's standard of work has dropped for some reason, then you would expect a Head to be supportive, to be saying: 'Oh, do you want to observe another teacher, I'll give you some time off teaching to work on this.' They certainly shouldn't be saying, in the first instance: 'I could take formal proceedings or I could give you a good reference.' That's the indication that it is

bullying, because a genuinely good, non-bullying Head would actually be trying to develop that person, to help them improve, and to keep them, as a valued member of the school staff. Not, 'Well – I could be really nasty, or you could go.'

In Emma's case the underhand comments, the off-the-cuff nasty phrases, the weak link bit, and the formal proceedings; well, this person is abusing their position of power. You know some Heads are totally and utterly ruthless in the sense of it's my way or no way if you don't like it. Really it's more about how you manage people, and getting the best out of people which is a real skill. A lot of people think that being a Manager or being a Head is about getting people to do it, to do what they're told, but there's ways and means of doing it, isn't there. It's maybe that some people think that they're showing weakness or they've got to be in control.

Headteachers who feel threatened

Andy had lots of experience and long service; he probably had good relationships with everyone and was often listened to, so that new Head probably came in and thought – well I'm the Head of this school – and maybe she felt threatened by him because he'd got such a lot of experience and such a good rapport with other colleagues and with the parents. But it's important to remember that not all Heads are like this. We have to make that point. Perhaps she felt she was under pressure: Heads are very isolated, they are under a number of pressures, nationally and also from Governors, about raising standards, about improving their attainment rates, around dealing with behaviour. And often they get no support from the Governors. It doesn't excuse the behaviour, but we do say to people who are being bullied, 'You don't know what pressure the Head's under, you don't know how stressed they are.' Sometimes it may be, if you've got a really good teacher, the Head actually feels intimidated and insecure, by having somebody who is very good. And they'd perhaps rather have somebody who doesn't challenge them as much.

A lot of Heads absolutely live in fear of the next Ofsted inspection, and all that pressure filters down. They interpret what they think Ofsted are going to be looking for, sometimes wrongly, so we get lots of teachers phoning up saying, 'I've got to produce these really detailed lesson plans,' as in Pauline's story, or, 'I'm being observed,' or, 'I've been told that Good isn't Good anymore and it's got to be Outstanding.' But if you go through the requirements for Ofsted or Teacher Standards, it doesn't say anywhere that things have got to be outstanding. There's lots of misinformation or interpretation by Heads about what they think is needed that's filtered down, and as that cascades down there's a lot of pressure being placed on teachers unnecessarily.

Ill-health

Health-wise, people don't want to be seen to be being affected. So you get people going into work when they really shouldn't be in, because they're too ill, which just increases the stress levels. And then someone can come in and say, 'Well, you're obviously not up to this.' They get into this vicious circle and won't stay off because someone might say they can't do the job, and if you stay off they're going to say you can't do it, so it goes round and round and round.

It's going to be an extremely difficult situation if you've been ill and had a breakdown as a result of school, and then tried to do something about it only to be told no, it's not our fault, it's your fault (as in Debbie's story). And it's very difficult for the Union at that stage, because what people are hoping is that everything will suddenly be all right, and they'll ease back into work. There's always an issue if you try and assist in that process by relieving people of some duties, as to whether that's seen as undermining or whether it's giving them extra time.

If a teacher has a breakdown or a stress related illness, it's sensible for an employer to refer them to Occupational Health. Ideally they are there to try and identify what the problem is, the root causes, and to take a view on that person's health, the prognosis of their condition, and recommend whether they're fit to return to work. If they are, then they must consider what support mechanisms need to be in place to facilitate their continued employment. So we wouldn't criticise an employer for referring a teacher to Occupational Health, because it is probably sensible in cases of a breakdown or stress.

There is the potential for people who have been bullied to pursue a personal injury claim, but the legal proof for that is immense. You've got to have a recognised mental health condition; it's not enough to be depressed or anxious. You've got to show that it was solely because of work and not, for example, because you were moving house or you were getting divorced. You also have to then show that that person acted in a way deliberately to damage your health, in a way that they knew would damage your health. And in order for them to know that, you will have to have written to them or said in some provable form that the way they were acting was making you ill. To fulfil all of those criteria is very difficult, particularly with people who've been bullied.

Too late

Unfortunately, some people come to us when they feel that they are at the end of the road, and that's a problem, they leave it a bit too late. And then they're off sick and it's just a case of, 'I'm not coming back to work again,' or, 'I just can't face it, it's never going to change.' So sometimes we're trying to talk them back from that and saying, 'Well look, there are actually things that could be done here.' The best result is when someone comes early and you've tried to look at the support of colleagues within the school. There is always a problem about evidence, and how you assess that, for example, 'It's your word against mine,' all that sort of thing. Our answer to that would be that if you're trying to make a claim to say they should be compensated, it might well be relevant to say what's the evidence, but there is a stage before that, which is not, 'Will I win a legal case,' but, 'Can I try and resolve this situation to the benefit of the member.'

Performance management

If your performance according to the line manager drops, you can be moved fairly rapidly through Capability Procedures. For teachers, contractually, employers should abide by the use of Capability. But if you've been teaching for a good number of years and then somebody starts to question your performance and your ability, that's a big knock to your confidence, particularly if you don't think there's any justification for it. Quite often that can be enough to push someone into absence, which may turn into long term absence, and which ultimately, if the employer's not willing to help them back into work, will turn into their departure from their employment.

In Emma's case in her performance management meeting everything was very positive, but the notes afterwards were not, and it's taken that the notes were the correct version. The problem is that anything that's said without a witness to verify it is open to interpretation, and each person is going to put their slant on the way they heard it. It's a real trap, because say somebody's been threatened with Competency in terms of management of pupil behaviour, you actually get to the point where the person who's being bullied can't really raise any issues about particularly difficult pupils in their class, or ask for help and support to deal with those pupils, because the answer will be that nobody else needs support, it's just you, you need to look at yourself. And it becomes a real Catch 22 situation for people.

Compromise agreements and references

Unfortunately we are often involved in negotiating an exit, where we basically get them a sum of money to terminate their employment, a Compromise Agreement, which I know is not really solving it but it allows them to look for another job and to get a reference. If a teacher is offered a Compromise Agreement, we would seek to maximise the level of compensation payable, and also seek an employment reference, so the teacher would be able to get another job.

If a teacher goes through the formal Capability process and they seem to by and large meet in full or in part all the various obligations, but at the end of it an employer still takes the view that that person is not capable of teaching to the performance that they need, then they can take them through a disciplinary procedure to dismiss them. What we find is, if you get to that point, by and large, employers will offer a Compromise Agreement, a deal, rather than sack them. And on the face of it, to the individual, rather than going through the disciplinary process, which is incredibly stressful, they may well think that that's the best option available to them. If it's just one person, and nobody else is prepared to stand up and be counted, then we might say to them: 'It might be in your best interests to leave the school.' Now that is just awful, as a trade Unionist, to give that advice, to negotiate a Compromise Agreement, but it's probably the best advice you can give in those circumstances. It's such a shame because the bully will then move onto somebody else. But it does get them the pay off and the reference.

In taking a Compromise Agreement the teacher foregoes all rights to challenge their employer in law, so they're giving away all their legal, statutory rights. A lot of people go out from the educational system in that way because, if there are issues of Capability that have ever been raised, they need to be included in the employment reference and that can make it very difficult for people to gain further employment. Their Capability in a particular school might have dropped for various reasons, such as the environment, the management style, even whether or not they got on with colleagues, but that doesn't make them a poor teacher per se. We've got loads of examples of people leaving poorly run schools and then excelling once they've got out.

Special relationships and conflict of interests

Sometimes it's not the hierarchical type of bullying, when the person who's doing it may feel that they've got the patronage of somebody. There was a Y1 teacher yesterday, in a two form intake school. She had been teaching for about 25 years, a very experienced teacher. But she was feeling quite intimidated and bullied by the NQT in the parallel class, in terms of how they should be doing things, producing their plans, what they should be working to, what subjects they should be doing, all this sort of thing. And she said, 'Well the problem that I feel that I have is that the NQT is very good friends with the Deputy Head.'

A similar situation recently occurred in a Secondary school where the Deputy Head is the sister of a member of the PE department. This teacher thought she was friends with the Head because her sister was the Deputy Head, and there was a serious conflict of interest going on within the PE department in that school. People felt really harassed by this woman and the Deputy Head, her sister, was refusing to see it. It made it very difficult for the Head because she had the Deputy Head on one side and the Deputy's sister there in the PE department on the other, and it was just spiralling out of control. In situations like that you have to have a strong management team who will step back and not be personally involved, and that wasn't happening there. If you've got a management who won't deal with it, then it leaves the member or person being bullied incredibly vulnerable, it eats away at them and they lose all their self-confidence.

6.2

Union Officials' Advice and Ways Forward

Looking at what can be done practically about these types of bullying, well we can ask questions such as: why are they being observed so much, what's the justification for this? Can you please explain why they are being observed so often? We need to question why teachers are being put under additional scrutiny, ask for details, just to try and pin it down a bit more. Because sometimes, with the drop-in observations and all that, what it does is it creates a general air of anxiety. And what you have to do is grab hold of that and get specifics, to try and reduce that general sense of something's not looking quite right here and I don't know what it is, and I'm a bit worried and I think my Head's watching me, and I'm not quite sure. Sometimes it's about can we try and pin it down so that people feel a bit more in control.

But bullying and intimidation gets spread within a school because teachers and other staff tend to put up with things. Members feeling bullied need to keep a record of every single communication they have with the Head: dates, times, witnesses, anybody who was there, the background to it, and a dossier of all of these incidents. We would use that dossier to have a conversation with the Head. Just having that conversation is a type of mediation before it all gets too serious. Often, when we make representations in that way, and say, 'Look. This is our record of things that have been happening.' It does make the Head sit up and think: 'Wow. I need to back off a bit here. This person's keeping a record.' So we'll get someone in to have a conversation, and we'll say, 'This is the teacher's experience. We have a record of this, because we've asked them to keep a record. This and that happened. We think he's being intimidated, harassed. At this point the teacher doesn't want to make a formal complaint but we say to you that if this continues we shall do this. And we're just putting it on record that this is an issue, that it's been raised.'

Our advice would be to send a friendly email after any meeting, saying, 'It was good to have met, I was pleased to have been able to raise blah blah,' you know, 'I look forward to your response,' or, 'Thank you for saying that you will do...' It's a point of reference, and it is evidence. This is what we can go back to.

If a member of staff has got a problem with the Head or a member of senior management, then doing something about that is very tricky. If you take a grievance procedure against your Head then it's incredibly difficult. We make it very clear on our website that, if this is where you find yourself, you must get advice before you do anything too hasty, because there's always that thing about what this could mean for you, and future relationships.

Employers are very reluctant to uphold grievances so we always say to a member, think about whether it is in your interests to formalise your concerns. That's not to say don't do anything, but once you start to move into grievance procedures the walls start to come up, and people start to defend their positions. It's usually more productive if you don't lodge a grievance but instead engage in a discussion, to seek to resolve it informally. If an employer upholds a grievance then in part they're admitting that things have broken down in a way that they shouldn't have done. And that gives the possibility for perhaps, say, a legal challenge.

It's not easy to get people to a place where they're prepared to stand up to their employer. We are powerless if our members won't support and defend their own position, but it certainly helps if they do it collectively. Our members want justice, they want the person to acknowledge that they've been bullied; they want them to know what they've put them through, which we completely understand. But quite often we might be able to get an agreement that they don't work with that person again, or maybe have a change of line manager, or a protocol for communication, or a Compromise Agreement to get them out of there. But we can't always get them the resolution that they want, that sense of personal satisfaction, and when someone's been severely traumatised, that is what they are looking for. If a Union can achieve that at the same time as getting the practical solutions, then that's fantastic, but I think a lot of the time that's not possible.

The view of a lot of members is that there must be some legal route, like 'an injunction' or 'a court order', that says, 'You have to stop bullying,' but there isn't, and it would be extremely difficult to try and put one in place. The problem with the law is that it's not really about justice or fairness, instead it's about giving people financial compensation for something that has damaged them. That level of proof in law is much higher than you could ever hope to achieve.

It's so frustrating when you don't get a group of members prepared to take a grievance together. You find yourself giving advice to the individual, which is kind of alien to what you would want to do as a trade Union rep, because you would want to say, 'Yes, we can fight this, we can sort it out.' As individuals they cannot produce witnesses and support from their colleagues to be able to successfully challenge things. If they take a grievance as an individual, quite often the person will be in a worse position because they'd tried to challenge it. We wouldn't, any longer, advise members , as individuals, to take out a grievance or a case against the Head because you just wouldn't be able to provide the evidence of what happened – it is amazing how many things can be passed off as, 'Oh, it wasn't meant in that way; that's a standard letter that people have to receive.' When each instance of bullying is taken as a one off incident it can be explained away – for the benefit of any panel of Governors. A collective approach is the only approach that's effective, because it does stop it.

Often bullying doesn't only happen to one person; it's something to do with the culture and the politics of the school. Our approach over the years has probably changed somewhat, to now, where we do try for it to be a collective response, because we think it's about relationships and the culture of the school as a whole. Collective action is always much more powerful than individual action: getting everyone to join in works if you've got a bullying Head. But some individuals don't want to do that because they don't want to be identified. Quite often, in these instances, Heads pick members off, go for the weakest member, which then gets them to withdraw or not sign up to it.

We get Union representatives who say, 'I've got 5 teachers in this school, who all feel bullied, but nobody's prepared to talk about it to anybody else. Sometimes they won't even let me say to other colleagues, you know, there are other people within the school who are feeling the same as you.' Even anonymously they won't allow that to be said because it's almost gone past that. So those are very difficult situations, because people are talking to you but you can't really do very much with it.

But a collective grievance, quite often that is very, very powerful. If you manage to do that, getting everyone to join in, if you've got a bullying Head, that works. This type of collective action has given teachers confidence to deal with issues such as bullying because they find that they've got the full workforce, or teachers, behind them, working together. Collective action is always much more powerful than individuals.

One union's approach to collective action

We developed a way of dealing with bullying, but really only when it comes from the Head or the SMT, of dealing with it as a collective issue, which got a number of people on board, prepared to give evidence. But we had to do it in a way that didn't identify people because in the main they were terrified of being identified. So we had meetings out of school hours, off-site, no names taken, and no notes taken. But what we did do was ask people to draft statements and give them to us as Unions. Initially, we went sometimes purely as a single Union, sometimes in cooperation with the other teaching Unions. We would go to the Head and say: these are issues that have been raised. We'd choose issues that could have come from anybody, so that nobody could be identified, and we'd give the Head an opportunity to change their ways, if you like. We'd give them maybe a half-term and then we'd ask our members if there'd been any change: there never was, really. And then we would start, we would contact the Chair of Governors, we'd work with the Local Authority, and we would put together evidence, again that didn't identify any particular person, but we had a questionnaire that we sent out.

The information we got from that was absolutely appalling, and to present a Chair of Governors with information that two thirds of your staff felt that they had been bullied, had seen the doctor because of stress related to it, that a couple of people might have been on suicide watch, from their doctor, how many of those people were intending to give up teaching altogether because of the treatment they'd had; we found that most Chairs of Governors would seek to deal with that. And in a number of cases we had Heads removed from their post without any further ado. I think in the end, for the ones that dealt with it very quickly, we'd produced fairly significant evidence, without identifying anybody, and what they basically said to Heads was:

this is the evidence that is going to be brought against you. We suggest that we do a deal. I have to say that the Heads who've gone, we know have gone with a good package and a good reference, which doesn't solve the problem completely. But there were a couple of instances out of the ones I've personally been involved with, where we went to an independent investigation and in some cases schools paid a firm of consultants, people who were involved with stress in work, through the Governors, or through the staffing committee In the 3 schools where we've gone through that process of having an independent investigation, the investigation has brought up so much evidence that there's never been a hearing against the Head. They have gone. It's very time-consuming, but it works. And it makes such a massive difference to how the school moves forward.

Now, where it hasn't been the Head and it's perhaps been a Head of faculty or department or somebody on the SMT, we've gone through the same process but it then has to be laid at the Head's door to tackle it. And it doesn't produce quite as dramatic a result. We've had such a remarkable effect, because Chairs of Governors and, in fact, the governing body, usually only get the view of the school that the Head gives them. And, for them to be presented with something in such stark contrast, I think shocks them and makes them act. Then they've got to manage the alleged bully in some way or other. And how do they deal with that? It's tricky but what we say is that the ethos in the school generally comes from the top. But we do appreciate that Heads have enormous pressures on them. They're doing a job now that they never trained, as a teacher, to do, and some of the schools are huge. Huge numbers, not just of teaching staff, but also support staff; if you've got over 100 teaching staff you've got, probably, over 100 support staff. And you do have to delegate to your SMT or to HODs, and I think in those circumstances it's not unusual for a Head to not appreciate. I think they should know what's being delivered in the school and they should know what the standard of teaching is, and how the school's moving forwards in terms of its results and so on, and everything else, but I don't think they could necessarily be expected to know the kind of interpersonal relationships and the kind of management style that goes on within what might be a very small department within that massive school

In undertaking this process of combating bullying our strategy would be:

- To work with other Unions representing both teaching and support staff.
- Send a short questionnaire to all members in the school where there are allegations of bullying so we can identify the number of teachers affected, the strength of feeling amongst them and the quantity and quality of evidence.
- Hold confidential joint Union meetings of members outside of the school day and away from the school, with invitations sent to members' home addresses.
- Make contact with the Local Authority, if it is a LA school, to apprise them of the situation.
- Meet with the Head to explain the teachers' concerns and agree actions to remedy the situation, with an agreed timescale for the bullying to stop.
- Present this in such a way that instances of bullying cannot be traced to an individual member.
- Inform the rep or members of the outcome of the discussion with the Head.
- Meet again with members to review the situation and to ask them to start drafting statements.
- If nothing has changed then meet with the Chair of Governors, and present the results of the questionnaire, taking care not to identify individual teachers or support staff.

SECTION THREE

What we know about the bullying of teachers now

Introduction

In Chapter 7 we revisit the research literature on bullying that we explored in Section 1. We summarise the experiences of the teachers, the views of Senior Managers and the advice of Union officials. We discuss organisational factors, such as leadership, staff support structures and accountability systems in schools in relation to workplace bullying.

We note in particular the effects of workplace bullying on the health and well-being of our volunteer teachers and the long-term costs to them. We then discuss possible ways forward, such as the provision of better support and training for senior leaders, emotional support for teachers, and the use of collective action.

Chapter 8 offers a brief 'two years on' update on what has happened to our volunteer teachers since they first told us about their experiences. Most are now teaching again in some capacity or other, more often than not in different schools; others have yet to recover their health.

7

CONCLUSION

7.1

Context, literature and findings

Our stories, responses and commentaries (Section 2) tell of individual teachers', Senior Managers' and Union officials' experiences of bullying in the school workplace. Our wider analysis (Section 1) illuminates and resonates with a particular historical context, that of the UK, and primarily English, education system in the years following the 1988 Education Reform Act (DES, 1988). There can be no doubt that both structural and systemic change has occurred in the intervening period, nor that such change has had a significant impact on the professional lives and workplace experiences of teachers in schools.

Those experiences are summarised here in Chapter 7, through articulation with prior research and the literature explored in Section 1. From our social scientific perspective we can say that, while all of our respondents are unique individuals and their stories and commentaries vary substantially in terms of specifics, we have also found that individual teacher experiences reflect many of the relationships we observed within the literature about workplace bullying.

Some of the changes precipitated by the 1988 Act relate to the literature on bullying and our teachers experiences. There has been:

- Increased prescription and reduced professional autonomy; increased levels of monitoring and accountability, both internal and external.

- Change in management, supervisory practices and responsibilities.
- Increased pressure and stress on both chalk-face teachers and their managers, including fragility in career structure and decreased pay security.

All of this has occurred alongside perennial incidences of change, such as new Heads being appointed and individual teachers moving schools.

Such factors undoubtedly shape the workplace environment and play a role in the bullying experienced by our teachers. But the relationship is complex. For example, some of the bullying took place in schools with a poor Ofsted rating, but there were also reports of bullying in schools where Ofsted ratings were good. Similarly, while there was a marked tendency for our teacher respondents to indicate that their being bullied commenced under a new Headteacher or senior line manager, a relationship supported in the literature (Illingworth, 2010; O'Moore et al., 1998), this clearly was not the case for all our teachers. Rather, we agree with Salin (2003, see Chapter 1, Fig. 1) that it is sensible to see many if not all of these change issues as potential triggers, aggravating factors or enablers, where motivations (i.e. rewards) for bullying might be found. For example, a new Headteacher might seek to save money on expensive experienced staff and replace them with cheaper NQTs or non-qualified staff with whom they might more readily establish their own educational philosophy or ways of doing things (Emma, Pauline, Andy, Maria, Debbie, Jo).

The change issues bulleted above have no doubt impacted on Senior Managers as much as they have on class-based teachers. Some of our Senior Managers and Union officials mentioned bullying of Headteachers during interview, but it is difficult to comment further on this because it was the teachers' rather than their managers' experiences of being bullied that were at the heart of this research. Nevertheless the literature indicates (Howard, 2011; French, 2009; Phillips, Sen & McNamee, 2007 & 2008) and our data confirm, that Senior Managers in schools do suffer high levels of stress and stress-related illness. They are accountable for their schools as teachers are accountable for their classes. Both groups have high demands placed upon them, both often feel isolated and fear losing their jobs if Ofsted's demands are not met, and both feel the need for better support.

There have been changes too in terms of school governance. Leading and managing schools has, post-ERA, post-LMS and post designation as Academies, become more difficult and more complex (Earley et al., 2012), with both Headteachers and their governors having to manage school administration, human resources (including staff appointments, promotions, performance-related pay, and CPD), and especially individual school budgets that now might cover all of the above if the schools are no longer under LA control. Where LAs control schools they can act as a support and buffer, talking to Heads and their staff, giving them advice on how to deal with staffing matters and economic resources, but Academy schools don't have that buffer; instead they have sponsors to whom they are responsible and there appears to be very little overt or formalised support for Senior Managers in Academy schools. However, as with Ofsted ratings, we found no indications that change from LA control to academy status might be a trigger for bullying behaviour.

The structural and systemic changes post-ERA link to four of the six HSE stressors (Cousins et al., 2004), namely change itself, demands made, degree of control, and factors associated with role. These, plus the last two HSE stressors, support and relationships, which are more likely to be directly influenced by school leaders and Senior Managers, were all found to affect the levels of stress and degrees of bullying experienced by staff. While the four external change pressures can be mediated and managed by Senior Managers, they can also be passed on – in terms of pressures on staff. Micro-management and overt (at times seemingly oppressive) supervision and monitoring of teachers can be the result. In many instances this is what we found from our teachers' individually reported experiences, alongside their need for support and positive relationships within their working environments.

While 'the system' is not directly responsible for individuals' experiences of bullying, or for individual bullies' specific actions, the post-ERA educational environment provided the context for an interaction between structures and processes from which bullying might result, hence it provided triggers (for organisational changes), alongside enablers (revised power structures and locations), and motivations (rewards/outcomes) (Salin, 2003). Schools have become workplaces where bullying by managers is more likely to happen (e.g. Beale & Hoel, 2011; Hauge et al., 2011; Skogstad, Matthiesen & Einarsen, 2007).

Bullying in the public sector is often seen in the research literature as a significant problem (particularly in the health and education sectors), but it also appears to be the least well understood or explained by sociologists, including Fevre et al's (2012) detailed study of 'Trouble at Work'.

Schools as organisations, and teachers as workers in them, do not readily fit with the conflict and class-based models used to address industrial relations. Senior managers and their staff (teachers) are not usually in direct conflict with each other on the basis of fundamentally different workplace interests and values, and teachers are not lowly placed unskilled workers with little autonomy (the most commonly bullied: Ferris et al., 2007). Although teacher autonomy has declined over the past 25 years they continue to be seen, within an industrial relations model, as skilled workers, with valued knowledge, working in professional workplace environments. Our teachers have demonstrated that they too are vulnerable to bullying behaviours, but the likely explanations for it are not helpfully illuminated by such traditional models.

Nevertheless, such understandings of workplace bullying do articulate with the views of our Union officials, particularly in terms of a desire to seek collective responses to bullies and bullying behaviours in schools. The extent of teacher unionisation would suggest this might be a reasonable way forward, yet it was rarely reported by our teachers, or Union officials, as the route that was actually taken.

Power: formal and informal

Formal power over teachers' work and employment is now vested in Senior school Managers, most usually the Headteacher, and it is they whom our teachers most frequently named as bullies. Ofsted judgements have enormous impact on schools and are implicated in the increase in teacher performance monitoring activity undertaken by Senior Managers. This monitoring is a legitimate enactment of formal, hierarchical power, but it is also an enactment that can be abused, as a great many of our teachers reported (see Emma, Debbie and Pauline's stories), and one which the post-ERA context serves to accentuate. As Webb and Vulliamy (1996: 448) argue, this climate of constant high stakes inspection encourages '...*Headteachers to be powerful and, if necessary, manipulative leaders...*'. Bentley et al., (2009: 30) explain that ...*excessive supervision can undermine autonomy and remove control over one's work, and may be a particularly powerful form of bullying because it increases feelings of powerlessness on the part of victims.*

Power, and its enactment in bullying behaviour, is also exercised informally. For example, on moving to a new school one of our experienced teachers was bullied by an NQT who had previously been a longstanding TA there; another teacher respondent reported being bullied by an administrator who appeared to her to be 'very close' to the Headteacher.

Teachers can clearly be subjected to bullying behaviours by a wide range of different people in their school workplaces, although our data do suggest that it is usually Senior Managers who bully, or who support (or ignore) bullying behaviour enacted by others.

Collective action

Our Union officials recommended collective action as their preferred way forward regarding their increasing casework of bullied teachers (Pauline and Union commentaries). Unionisation, which facilitates collective action, was strong amongst our teachers, and structural issues, such as pay and conditions, were regularly addressed in this way. However this was not the case with bullying. Our teachers spoke about 'divide and rule', fearful staffrooms, a reluctance to put 'heads above parapets' (see Jenny, Andy and Pauline's stories), and managers not knowing how to deal with reports and complaints of bullying appropriately (Debbie). Any public challenge or confrontation worsened rather than improved their situations (Andy, Emma).

While on occasion reported to be sympathetic, aware and supportive of individual victims, our teachers said that their teacher colleagues' actions tended more towards self protection, and that they rarely spoke out or stood up for them. Fear of becoming the bully's next target, or for their own jobs or careers, generally took precedence. And unfortunately, in a great many incidences, our bullied teachers chose to leave, often with a Compromise Agreement that ensured a reference, rather than to stay and fight, either through employment tribunals or the more remote possibility of collective action. Most commonly our bullied teachers felt they had to cope with their problems in isolation, and repair or recover themselves alone or with family support (Pauline, Jo, Maria, Andy).

Capability Procedures and Compromise Agreements

Problems surrounding the nature and extent of Capability issues in schools are recognised in the literature (e.g. Morrell et al., 2010), and evidenced in our data. Rather than organising collective action our Union officials usually found themselves dealing with members on long term sick leave, threatened with CPs, or supporting staff through CAs or towards an early retirement. For any and all of this they required teachers to collect, keep and provide documentation, written records of conversations, interactions and events that evidenced the bullying behaviours.

Bullies, especially Senior Managers, frequently raised questions regarding teacher Capability, and often threatened to instigate CPs (see Emma and Debbie's stories). Like Earnshaw et al., (2002), we found that the majority of our teachers who were subject to CPs resigned without them being completed. There were a variety of reasons for this. While CPs are intended to be supportive in terms of improving a teacher's practice, that is not how they were conducted or experienced by our teachers. Clarity about aims and actions were rare, actual support rarer, with teachers, Senior Managers and Union officials seeing CPs ultimately as a tool to remove the teacher (or even more frequently prompting the teachers to remove themselves in order to salvage whatever might be left of their careers).

We found that CPs were threatened, or used, against many teachers whose teaching had historically been assessed as good or very good, and against older or long serving teachers, who might be expensive to employ, and/or whose competence or experience led their bully to feel threatened by them (for example, Emma). And many of our teachers had a strong sense that their bully's actions were designed to make them leave.

Few teachers sought redress through their schools' governing bodies, which were generally thought to support Senior Managers, largely uncritically; outcomes of complaints and tribunals appeared to them to be determined, in many cases, prior to any hearing, something that Wilkins (2014) suggests is not uncommon: '...a lot of decisions are sewn up in advance of full governing meetings'. This is both disappointing and disempowering for bullied teachers because legally, and in the first instance, it is the governing body to which they should appeal if they believe they have been unfairly treated. It is telling that most of our teachers declined to take this route. As independent scrutinisers of complaints, Capability or disciplinary issues, our teachers deemed their school governors to be lacking.

CPs and CAs do not necessarily mean that a teacher is inadequate. In most instances where CAs were sought or accepted by our teachers it was primarily to secure an employment reference. However, CA guidance suggests that where issues of Capability have been raised then they need to be included in the reference, which in turn makes it difficult to get further employment. Several of our teachers believed they were offered CAs in order to get them to leave.

Bullying and ill-health

A strong relationship between bullying and teacher ill-health was found within our data. Other research (for example: Neilsen & Einarsen, 2012; Cooper, Hoel & Faragher, 2004) suggests that pre-existing health problems can make people more vulnerable to bullying and more likely to report it. However, while few of our teachers had pre-existing health problems all but one reported serious mental health problems such as anxiety and depression after being bullied. For the majority of our sample, mental health problems were a consequence of, not a precursor to, being bullied.

Figure 4 (see Chapter 3, but repeated below for ease of reading) illustrates the relationship between bullying and ill-health for our teachers, and the outcomes, at the time of interviews in 2012, in terms of their teaching careers.

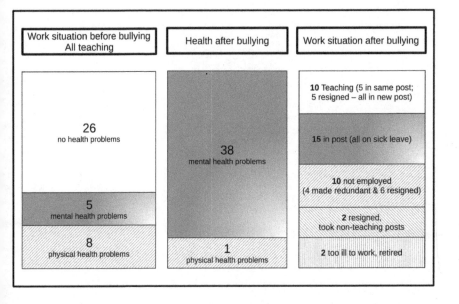

Figure 4: Thirty nine teacher accounts of work situation in 2012 before and after bullying

Figure 4 also indicates loss of these teachers from the teaching profession at the time of interview in 2012. Only 10 were still teaching (5 in the same school, 5 in new schools) while 15 others were on long-term sick leave and 14 had left teaching, mainly as a result of unresolved mental health problems when teaching.

The teachers' stories show how they were treated unfairly, humiliated, undermined and threatened, while Figure 4 (above) shows that such treatment made all but one of them ill, or more ill, as a result! As in Giga, Hoel and Lewis's (2008b) research, many of our teachers suffered extensive periods of sick leave and impaired performance. Such treatment can have long term negative effects including the loss of competent and experienced teachers to the profession. None of this is helpful to schools as organisations because sick leave is a financial burden, and high staff turnover is disruptive.

What to do about teacher bullying: Work together or carry on crying in cupboards?

No doubt there are many underlying and generic problems related to workplace bullying, including the bullying of teachers in schools. However we believe the post-ERA context in which teachers currently work can only exacerbate them. Like others before us (Di Martino, Hoel & Cooper, 2003) we cannot identify a clear profile of either bullies or targets within our data, although the perpetrators were more likely to be Senior Managers, often in a new post, and the victims, often several of them in each school (e.g. Jenny, Pauline, Andy), and sometimes unbeknown to each other, tended to suffer and respond individually rather than collectively to the experience. That is a heavy burden to bear, and its cost to the individual teacher's health is huge.

While some of our teachers agreed with Union officials that collective action was in principle a sensible way forward, and potentially effective, there was a strong element of fear – about references, damaged careers, reprisals and intimidation – strong enough to seriously inhibit the mutual advocacy of peers that is required for collective action to be successfully attempted. Support from fellow teachers and TAs for complaints about bullying exists in our data, but it was a rare occurrence. Most kept their heads 'below the parapet', fearing it might be them next. Our Union officials suggest that where collective action has been undertaken by teachers with Union support it has been successful.

Despite their formal role in complaints procedures, school governors were not trusted by our teacher volunteers to act independently of Heads and Senior Managers. Independent arbitration was the most recommended way forward by our teachers, something separate from, and independent of, the schools in which they were being bullied. The GTCE might once have been developed appropriately to fill this role, but it was abolished in March 2012 and a new independent body to which teachers might turn is much needed.

Overall our data and the teachers' stories suggest that a good deal of the bullying may be triggered by a practical desire to reduce costs – by removing older more expensive staff (Emma, Pauline), or those who are likely to need considerable support and resources to be provided by the school (Debbie). Equally, a good deal of the bullying appears to be triggered by high rather than low levels of competence and experience, with newly powerful (sometimes much younger) Senior Managers feeling threatened by the traditional and professional challenges or constructive advice offered by long serving and respected peers (Andy).

We do believe that schools aspire to be caring environments that support and develop their teachers but it is an aspiration undermined by excessive accountability, inspection and ranking, which increases stress amongst teachers and their Senior Managers. The bullying reported here took place at the level of individual schools, but schools, their leaders and the teachers in them are also being bullied by outside bodies, such as government agencies, especially with set performance targets that might be either unachievable or which cannot be achieved without placing significant stress and pressure on the schools and their teaching staff.

Regarding the mental health of teachers, Rothi, Leavey and Loewenthal (2010: 43-44) make two recommendations with which we concur:

- that the cumulative impact of accountability systems in schools be reviewed;
- that high quality support and training for senior leaders, including the emotional support of colleagues, needs to be established.

This might go some way towards addressing the unacceptable behaviour, high workload, unsupportive workplaces and bad management practices that our teachers described to us. Consigning threatening behaviour, such as Ofsted's current Head, Sir Michael Wilshaw's promise (2012, NAHT's National Conference) of '*an unforgiving climate for inspection*' to the dustbin would also be helpful.

Our teachers spoke in detail about their experiences, despite the very upsetting nature of some of these. As painful as some of the interviews were, these teachers believed that the problem of workplace bullying should be made public. They willingly gave their time, and opened up the pain of being bullied into ill-health to two stranger researchers in order that their stories be told, and that others might know what is happening in their schools. They actively keep in touch; most of them regularly updating us on their personal and professional progress, which we hope, for them, is towards a full recovery. Their participation in this research could be seen as a form of resistance (Fahie & Devine, 2012; Lutgen-Sandvik, 2006), and one of the few positive strategies available to them for fighting back – one has even published her own book about her experiences!

In Stephen Ball's terms (2003: 215) the current performative requirement in education portends inner conflict, inauthenticity and resistance amongst teachers (and their mangers), leading them to '*organise themselves as a response to targets, indicators and evaluations... and live an existence of calculation*'. For some that is, as we have seen, a bullied existence, and one that is not worth living! Teachers crying in cupboards is an unhealthy, unrewarding and damaging scenario for everyone – government, school mangers, teachers and ultimately the education of all our children.

8

TWO YEARS ON

Where are they now?

Well a lot has happened in the two years since our initial data collection. Here we give a brief update on the personal and professional outcomes for 38 of our 39 teacher interview respondents.

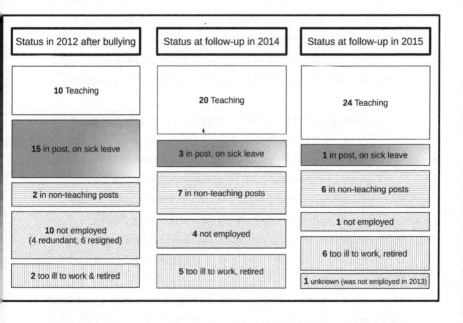

Figure 5: Teacher accounts of status in 2012 and at follow up in 2014 & 2015

This figure updates the information given earlier in Figure 4. Two years on from interview, in December 2014, we knew that there had been some significant developments and by the end of January 2015 we had heard from all but one of our volunteers. Twenty five of our 39 teachers were teaching again in some capacity or other (full-time, part-time or supply work, although one was on sick leave) mostly in different schools from where the bullying had taken place; 6 had changed career, although 4 of these were in teaching–related work (TA or adult training); 1 remained too ill to work and was now not emplyed and living on disability allowance, and 6 had retired, 3 as a result of their continuing ill-health. Only one remains unknown.

There is a noticeable and important difference here: two years on from our initial data analysis 15 more teachers had returned to teaching in some capacity or other. Seven of these had taken a Compromise Agreement after being threatened with Capability Procedures and all now report doing well in their new schools.

It's not easy for Senior Managers, and we have no wish to damn them all with our teachers' stories. They face similar pressures:

> …ultimately I'm going to be judged… I've got to get a good 75% of my staff to be Good to Outstanding. So if I've got 25% who are Satisfactory to Inadequate then that means I've got to assist that 25% in moving on. And that's really difficult when some people actually say well, and I've had it myself, somebody said, 'Well I'm satisfactory, that's good enough' And if everybody said that, we'd be a failing school
> (Primary Headteacher)

Our email updates suggest that slowly but surely more and more bullied teachers are returning to teaching – definitely a bit older, no doubt wiser, and hopefully stronger, to face those ever increasing pressures in the workplace that they all love – schools.

In the last Literacy classroom observation my teaching was judged as outstanding. I was tempted to send a copy to my previous Head!

I am far more confident in my ability, more assertive and less prepared to tolerate unacceptable behaviour from anyone. I laugh daily, work with a great team and a superb Head who cares about her staff.

I am not the person I once was and probably will not be again. Although now employed in a rewarding, intellectually challenging and valuable new role I still miss teaching very much.

Appendix

1. Education Support Partnership (TSN) e-newsletter request for participants

Researchers from the University of Hertfordshire would like to hear about teachers' personal experiences of workplace bullying. We are seeking volunteers to help us with the book we are producing about workplace bullying of teachers in schools. We are asking teacher volunteers to take part in one-to-one private conversations where you can tell us in complete privacy about your experiences of workplace bullying or, if preferred, to complete a very short survey form telling us about your experiences. We hope to hear from both primary and secondary school teachers from many different levels within schools. We would very much like to hear both from those who have experienced bullying and also from those in senior positions who have to deal with allegations of workplace bullying within their school. The experiences you tell us about will be available only to the researchers. Nothing will be reported in a way that lets people identify you or your workplace. We will not share personal information with anyone else. We value your opinions and suggestions and your response could have a positive influence on teachers' experiences in the current educational environment. If you have an interesting experience to relay, and would like to participate by talking to us face-to-face please contact us by clicking on the link below. No travelling will be involved; the researchers will travel to you. One of the researchers will contact you early in the New Year.

2. Examples of Bullying Behaviours

- Sarcasm, jokes, insults, or innuendo to mock, demean or belittle, in public or private.
- Attacks on personal characteristics, professional standing and rumour mongering.
- Undue and relentless criticism of work, fault-finding, undermining by being given trivial tasks to do.
- Work overload and task setting that undermines job performance, being set up to fail.
- Responsibility increased but authority diminished, stolen credit and inappropriate blame.
- Ignoring or excluding individuals from activities, withholding information, sidelining, ostracising.
- Excessive and unreasonable supervision, monitoring and criticism about minor things.
- Threats of and abuse of disciplinary and competency procedures.
- Obstructing professional development, training and promotion.
- Withholding of work responsibilities and recognition of performance.
- Refusal or ignoring of reasonable requests, being given demeaning/ menial tasks, de-skilling.

3. Some findings from the teachers interviewed

i) Their age range

Age range (Years)	Primary level	Secondary level	All teachers
26-35	4	2	6
36-45	9	4	13
46-55	6	8	14
56-65	5	1	6

ii) Their years of teaching experience

Years teaching experience	Primary level	Secondary level	All teachers
NQT only	2	0	2
Less than 5	2	0	2
5-10	6	5	11
11-20	5	3	8
21-30	6	6	12
31 or more	3	1	4

iii) Their responsibilities

Responsibilities	Primary level	Secondary level	All teachers
Headteacher	1	0	1
Assistant Head	0	1	1
HOD	0	3	3
HOY	0	1	1
SMT	7	1	8
AST	1	0	1
Coordinator	6	0	1
Misc responsibilities	2	3	5
None	7	6	13

iv) Bullying behaviour described by teachers

Bullying behaviour	Primary level	Secondary level	All teachers
Undermining	19	13	32
Verbal abuse	19	12	31
Unreasonable objectives	16	12	28
Exclusion	17	9	26
Persistent criticism	15	9	24
Competency (capability)	13	4	17
Blocking	6	1	7
Physical assault	0	1	1

*Total is greater than the total number of teachers as they usually cited a number of different behaviours.

v) Bullies identified by teachers

Workplace bully	Primary	Secondary	All teachers
Headteacher only	13	2	15
Headteacher and a member of senior management	5	6	11
Senior management only	2	5	7
Other staff (with support of senior management)	3	2	5
Governor	1	0	1

vi) Age-range of schools where bullying took place

School level	n
Primary	22*
Secondary	15

* Four teachers volunteered from two schools

References

Adamson, J., Owen, K. & Dhillon, S. (2011) *The experience of prejudice-related bullying and harassment amongst teachers and head teachers in schools.* Birmingham: NASUWT. (11/04017).

Addison, R. & Brundrett, M. (2008) Motivation and demotivation of teachers in primary schools: the challenge of change. *Education 3-13.* 36 (1). p.79-94.

Aelterman, A., Engels, N., Petegem K. & van Verhaeghe J.P. (2007) The well-being of teachers in Flanders: the importance of a supportive school culture. *Educational Studies.* 33 (3). p.285-297.

Agervold, M. (2009) The significance of organizational factors for the incidence of bullying. *Scandinavian Journal of Psychology.* 50 (3). p.267–276.

Agervold, M. & Mikkelsen, E. G. (2004) Relationships between bullying, psychosocial work environment and individual stress reactions. *Work and Stress.* 18 (4). p.336-351.

Alterman, T., Luckhaupt, S. E., Dahlhamer, J. M., Ward, B. W., & Calvert, G. M. (2013) Job insecurity, work-family imbalance, and hostile work environment: Prevalence data from the 2010 National Health Interview Survey. *American Journal of Industrial Medicine.* 56 (6). p.660–669.

Armstrong, P. (2011) Budgetary bullying. *Critical Perspectives on Accounting.* 22 (7). p.632–643.

ATL. (2011) *A quarter of education staff have been bullied by colleagues.* Press release, ATL Annual Conference. [Online] April 20th. Available from: www.atl.org.uk.

Avolio, B. J., Bass, B. M., & Jung, D. I. (1999) Re-examining the components of transformational and transactional leadership using Multifactor Leadership. *Journal of Occupational and Organizational Psychology.* 72 (4). p.441–462.

Baillien, E. & De Witte, H. (2009) Why is Organizational Change Related to Workplace Bullying? Role Conflict and Job Insecurity as Mediators. *Economic and Industrial Democracy*. 30 (3). p.348–371.

Ball, S.J. (2003) The teacher's soul and the terrors of performativity. *Journal of Education Policy*. 18 (2). p.215-228.

Bass, B. M. (1997) Does the transactional–transformational leadership paradigm transcend organizational and national boundaries? *American Psychologist*. 52 (2). p.130-139.

Bass, B. M. & Riggio, R. E. (2006) *Transformational leadership*. 2nd Edition. Mahwah, New Jersey: Lawrence Erlbaum Associates .

Beale, D. & Hoel, H. (2010) Workplace bullying, industrial relations and the challenge for management in Britain and Sweden. *European Journal of Industrial Relations*. 16 (2). p.101–118.

Beale, D. & Hoel, H. (2011) Workplace bullying and the employment relationship: exploring questions of prevention, control and context. *Work, Employment & Society*. 25 (1). p.5–18.

Beck, J. (2009) Appropriating professionalism: restructuring the official knowledge base of England's 'modernised' teaching profession. *British Journal of Sociology of Education*. 30(1). p.3-14.

Bentley, T., Catley, B., Cooper-Thomas, H., Gardner, D., O'Driscoll, M. & Trenberth, L. (2009)
Understanding Stress and Bullying in New Zealand Workplaces. Final report to OH&S Steering Committee. [Online] Available *from:* www.massey.ac.nz/massey/fms/.../2010/04/.../Bentley-et-al-report.pdf.

Berthelsen, M., Skogstad, A., Lau, B. & Einarsen, S. (2011) Do they stay or do they go?: A longitudinal study of intentions to leave and exclusion from working life among targets of workplace bullying. *International Journal of Manpower*. 32 (2). p.178–193.

Billehøj, H. (2007) *Report on the ETUCE Survey on Teachers' Work-related Stress*. European Trade Union Committee for Education. [Online] Available from: http://teachersosh.homestead.com/Publications/DraftReport_WRS_EN.pdf.

Bird, R. (2008) Does a new head-teacher spell trouble for staff? *Secondary Headteacher*. May.

Blasé, J., Blasé, J. & Du, F. (2008) The mistreated teacher: a national study. *Journal of Educational Administration*. 46(3). p.263–301.

Blaug, R., Kenyon, A. & Lekhi, R. (2007) *Stress at Work*. London: The Work Foundation. [Online] Available from: http://www. theworkfoundation.com/downloadpublication/report/69_69_stress_at_work.pdf

Bottery, M. (2001) Globalisation and the UK Competition State: No room for transformational leadership in education? *School Leadership & Management*. 21(2). p.199–218.

Branch, S., Ramsay, S. & Barker, M. (2007) Contributing factors to workplace bullying by staff – an interview study. *Journal of Management & Organization*. 13(3). p.264–281.

Bricheno, P. & Thornton, M. (2006) *The Voices Of The Disenchanted: Why Teachers Leave Teaching*. Paper presented at BERA, University of Warwick, 6-9 September.

Bright, T. & Ware, N. (2003) *Were You Prepared?* Findings from a National Survey of Head teachers. Summary Practitioner Enquiry Report. Nottingham: NCSL.

Bristow, M., Ireson, G. & Coleman, A. (2007) *A life in the day of a head teacher: a study of practice and well-being*. [Online] Available from: http://dera.ioe.ac.uk/7066/2/ download%3Fid=17101&filename=a-life-in-the-day-of-a-headteacher.pdf.

Brown M. & Ralph S. (2002) Teacher stress and school improvement. *Improving Schools*. 5(2). p.55-65.

Bubb, S., Earley, P. & Totterdell, M. (2005) Accountability and Responsibility: 'rogue' school leaders and the induction of new teachers in England. *Oxford Review of Education*. 31(2). p.255-272.

Bush, T. & Glover, D. (2003) *School leadership: Concepts and evidence*. [Online] Available from: http://dera.ioe.ac.uk/5119/2/dok217-eng-School_Leadership_Concepts_and_Evidence.pdf.

Butt R, & Retallick J. (2002) Professional well-being and learning: a study of administrator-teacher workplace relationships. *Journal of Educational Enquiry*. 3(1). p.17-34.

Carter, M., Thompson, N., Crampton, P., Morrow, G., Burford, B., Illing, J. & Gray, C. (2013) Workplace bullying in the UK NHS:

a questionnaire and interview study on prevalence, impact and barriers to reporting. *BMJ Open.* 3(6). [Online] Available from: http://www.ncbi.nlm.nih.gov/pmc/articles/PMC3686220/. [Accessed: 3rd November 2015].

Case, P., Case, C. & Catling, S. (2000) Please Show You're Working: a critical assessment of the impact of OFSTED inspection on primary teachers. *British Journal of Sociology of Education.* 21(4). p.605-621.

Cemaloglu, N. (2007) The Exposure Of Primary School Teachers To Bullying: An Analysis Of Various Variables. *Social Behaviour & Personality: An International Journal.* 35(6). p.789-802.

Cemaloglu, N. (2011) Primary principals' leadership styles, school organizational health and workplace bullying. *Journal of Educational Administration.* 49(5). p.495–512.

Cerit, Y. (2013) The Relationship between Paternalistic Leadership and Bullying Behaviours towards Classroom Teachers. *Theory and Practice of Educational Sciences.* 13(2). p. 847-851.

Charmaz, K. (2006) *Constructing Grounded Theory.* London: Sage Publications.

Cooper, C. L., Hoel, H. & Faragher, B. (2004) Bullying is detrimental to health, but all bullying behaviours are not necessarily equally damaging. *British Journal of Guidance & Counselling.* 32(3). p.367–387.

Crotty, M. (1998) *The Foundations of Social Research.* Sydney: Allen and Unwin.

Cousins , R., MacKay, C. J., Clarke, S. D., Kelly, C., Kelly, P. J. & McCaig, R. H. (2004) "Management Standards" work-related stress in the UK: practical development. *Work & Stress.* 18(2). p.113–136.

Cunningham, I., James, P. & Dibben, P. (2004) Bridging the gap between rhetoric and reality: line managers and the protection of job security for ill workers in the modern workplace. *British Journal of Management.* 15(3). p.273–290.

Day, C. & Sammons, P. (2013) *Successful leadership.* [Online] Available from: http://cdn.cfbt.com/~/media/cfbtcorporate/files/research/2013/r-successful-leadership-2013.pdf.

Day, C., Harris, A. & Hadfield, M. (2001) Challenging the Orthodoxy of Effective School Leadership. *International Journal of Leadership in Education.* 4(1). p.39–56.

De Wet, C. (2010) The reasons for and the impact of principal-on-teacher bullying on the victims' private and professional lives. *Teaching and Teacher Education*. 26(7). p.1450–1459.

De Wet, C. (2014) Educators' understanding of workplace bullying. *South African Journal of Education*. 34(1). p.1–16.

Dean, C., Dyson, A., Gallannaugh, F., Howes A. & Raffo C. (2007) *Schools, governors and disadvantage*. York: Joseph Rowntree Foundation. [Online] Available from: http://www.jrf.org.uk/bookshop/eBooks/1994-schools-governors-disadvantage.pdf.

Department for Education (DFE). (2013) School Teachers' Pay and Conditions Document 2013, and Guidance on School Teachers' Pay and Conditions. [Online] Available from: https://www.gov.uk/.../system/.../130806_2013_stpcd_master_final.pdf. [Accessed: 3rd November 2015].

Department for Education (DFE). (2014) *Teachers' workload diary survey 2013: Research Report*. London: Department for Education. (TNS BMRB [2014] Reference DFE-RR316).

Department for Education and Science (DES). (1967) *Children and their Primary Schools: A Report of the Central Advisory Council for Education*. London: HMSO.

Department for Education and Science (DES). (1987) *The National Curriculum 5-16: A Consulatative Document*. London: HMSO.

Department for Education and Science (DES). (1988) The Education Reform Act 1988. London: HMSO.

Di Martino, V., Hoel, H. & Cooper, C. L. (2003) *Preventing violence and harassment in the workplace*. Dublin: European Foundation for the Improvement of Living and Working Conditions/ Luxemburg: Office for Official Publications of the European Communities.

Djurkovic, N., McCormack, D. & Casimir, G. (2006) Neuroticism and the Psychosomatic Model of Workplace Bullying. *Journal of Managerial Psychology*. 21(1). p.73–88.

Djurkovic, N., McCormack, D. & Casimir, G. (2008) Workplace bullying and intention to leave: the moderating effect of perceived organisational support. *Human Resource Management Journal*. 18(4). p.405–422.

Earley, P., Higham, R., Allen, R., Allen, T., Howson, J., Nelson, R., Rawar, S., Lynch, S., Morton, L., Mehta, P. & Sims, D. (2012) *Review of the school leadership landscape.* Nottingham: National College for School Leadership.

Earley, P., Weindling, D., Bubb, S. & Glenn, M. (2009) Future leaders: the way forward? *School Leadership & Management.* 29(3). p.295–306.

Earnshaw, J., Ritchie, E., Marchington, L., Torrington, D. & Hardy, S. (2002) *Best practice in undertaking teacher capability procedures.* Manchester School of Management, UMIST Manchester: Department for Education and Skills. (Research Report No. RR312).

Einarsen, S. (1999) The Nature and Causes of Bullying at Work. *International Journal of Manpower.* 20(1/2). p.16-27.

Einarsen, S. (2000) Harassment and bullying at work: a review of the Scandinavian approach. *Aggression and Violent Behavior.* 5(4). p.379–401.

Einarsen, S. & Raknes, B. (1997) Harassment at work and the victimization of men. *Violence and Victims.* 12(3). p.247–263.

Einarsen, S. & Skogstad, A. (1996) Bullying at work: Epidemiological findings in public and private organizations. *European Journal of Work and Organizational Psychology.* 5(2). p.185–201.

Einarsen, S., Aasland, M. S. & Skogstad, A. (2007) Destructive leadership behaviour: A definition and conceptual model. *The Leadership Quarterly.* 18(3). p.207–216.

Einarsen, S., Hoel, H. & Notelaers, G. (2009) Measuring exposure to bullying and harassment at work: Validity, factor structure and psychometric properties of the Negative Acts Questionnaire-Revised. *Work & Stress.* 23(1). p.24–44.

Einarsen, S., Hoel, H., Zapf, D. & Cooper, C. (2011) The concept of bullying at work: the European tradition. In Einarsen, S., Hoel, H., Zapf, D. & Cooper, C. (eds.). *Bullying and Harassment in the Workplace: Developments in Theory, Research, and Practice.* 2nd Edition. Florida: CRC Press, Taylor and Francis Group.

Einarsen, S., Hoel, H., Zapf, D. & Cooper, C.L. (2003) The concept of bullying at work. In Einarsen, S., Hoel, H., Zapf, D. & Cooper, C. (eds.). *Bullying and Emotional Abuse in the Workplace:*

International Perspectives in Research and Practice. London: Taylor and Francis.

Einarsen, S., Raknes, B.I. & Matthiesen, S.B. (1994) Bullying and harassment at work and their relationships to work environment quality. An exploratory study. *European Work and Organisational Psychologist.* 4(4). p.381-401.

Ertureten, A., Cemalcilar, Z. & Aycan, Z. (2013) The Relationship of Downward Mobbing with Leadership Style and Organizational Attitudes. *Journal of Business Ethics.* 116(1). p.205–216.

Evans, L. (2011) The "shape" of teacher professionalism in England: professional standards, performance management, professional development and the changes proposed in the 2010 White Paper. *British Educational Research Journal.* 37(5). p.851–870.

Fahie, D. & Devine, D. (2014) The Impact of Workplace Bullying on Primary School Teachers and Principals. *Scandinavian Journal of Educational Research.* 58(2). p.235-252.

Ferris, G. R., Zinko, R., Brouer, R. L., Buckley, M. R. & Harvey, M. G. (2007) Strategic bullying as a supplementary, balanced perspective on destructive leadership. *The Leadership Quarterly.* 18(3). p.195–206.

Fetherston, T. & Lummis, G. (2012) Why Western Australian secondary teachers resign. *Australian Journal of Teacher Education.* 37(4). [Online] Available from: http://dx.doi.org/10.14221/ajte.2012v37n4.1. [Accessed: 3rd November 2015].

Fevre, R., Lewis, D., Robinson, A. & Jones, T. (2011) Insight into ill-treatment in the workplace: patterns, causes and solutions. *ESRC Report.* [Online] Available from: http://www.cf.ac.uk/socsi/resources/insight11.pdf.

Fevre, R., Lewis, D., Robinson, A. & Jones, T. (2012) *Trouble At Work.* London: Bloomsbury Academic.

Fevre, R., Nichols, T., Prior, G. & Rutherford, I. (2009) *Fair Treatment at Work Report: findings from the 2008 survey.* Department for Business, Innovation and Skills. [Online] Available from: https://www.gov.uk/government/uploads/system/uploads/attachment_data/file/192191/09-P85-fair-treatment-at-work-report-2008-survey-errs-103.pdf.

Fevre, R., Robinson, A., Lewis, D. & Jones, T. (2013) The ill-treatment of employees with disabilities in British workplaces. *Work, Employment & Society.* 27(2). p.288–307.

Foster, D. (2007) Legal obligation or personal lottery?: Employee experiences of disability and the negotiation of adjustments in the public sector workplace. *Work, Employment & Society.* 21(1). p.67–84.

Foucault, M. (1998) *The History of Sexuality, Vol.1: The will to knowledge.* London: Penguin.

Foucault, M. (2002) *Power. Essential works of Foucault 1954-1984. Vol.3.* London: Penguin.

Fox, S. & Stallworth, L. E. (2010) The battered apple: An application of stressor-emotion-control/support theory to teachers' experience of violence and bullying. *Human Relations.* 63(7). p.927–954.

French, S. (2009) *The NAHT Work-Life Balance Survey 2008-9.* Twenty4-7 Survey. Keele: Centre for Industrial Relations Institute for Public Policy & Management, Keele University.

Galanaki, E. & Papalexandris, N. (2013) Measuring workplace bullying in organisations. *The International Journal of Human Resource Management.* 24(11). p.2107–2130.

Galton, M. & Macbeath, J. (2008) *Teachers Under Pressure.* London: Sage.

Galton, M. & MacBeath, J. with Charlotte Page and Susan Steward. (2002) *A Life in Teaching? The Impact of Change on Primary Teachers' Working Lives.* A Report commissioned by the National Union of Teachers concerning the workloads in Primary Schools. London: NUT.

General Teaching Council for England (GTC). (2011) *Removing barriers, promoting opportunities Shaping the future for teachers with disabilities in England.* [Online]. Available from: http://www.gtce.org.uk/media_parliament/news_comment/remove_barriers_rpt030511/. [Accessed: 3rd November 2015].

Gholamzadeh, D. & Khazaneh, A. T. (2012) *Surveying The Relationships Between Leadership Styles, Organizational Health And Workplace Bullying.* Journal of Global Strategic Management, 12. [Online]. Available from: http://isma.info/uploads/files/005-surveying-the-relationships-between-leadership-styles--organizational-health-and-workplace-bullying.pdf. [Accessed: 3rd November 2015].

Giga, S. I., Hoel, H. & Lewis, D. (2008a) *A Review of Black and Minority Ethnic (BME) Employee Experiences of Workplace Bullying.* Research Commissioned by the Dignity at Work Partnership: A Partnership Project Funded Jointly by Unite the Union and the Department for Business, Enterprise and Regulatory Reform. Manchester UK: University of Bradford.

Giga, S. I., Hoel, H. & Lewis, D. (2008b) *The Costs of Workplace Bullying.* Research Commissioned by the Dignity at Work Partnership: A Partnership Project Funded Jointly by Unite the Union and the Department for Business, Enterprise and Regulatory Reform. Manchester UK: University of Bradford.

Glasø, L., Matthiesen, S. B., Nielsen, M. B. & Einarsen, S. (2007) Do targets of workplace bullying portray a general victim personality profile? *Scandinavian Journal of Psychology.* 48(4). p.313–319.

Glatter, R. (2012) Persistent Preoccupations: The Rise and Rise of School Autonomy and Accountability in England. *Educational Management Administration & Leadership.* 40(5). p.559–575.

Grenville-Cleave, B. & Boniwell, I. (2012) Surviving or thriving? Do teachers have lower perceived control and well-being than other professions? *Management in Education.* 26(1). p.3–5.

Griva, K. & Joekes, K. (2003) UK teachers under stress. *Psychology and Health.* 18(4). p.457-471.

Gu, Q. & Day, C. (2013) Challenges to teacher resilience: conditions count. *British Educational Research Journal.* 39(1). p.22-44.

Hansen, Å. M., Hogh, A., Persson, R., Karlson, B., Garde, A. H. & Ørbæk, P. (2006) Bullying at work, health outcomes, and physiological stress response. *Journal of Psychosomatic Research.* 60(1). p.63–72.

Hargreaves, L., Cunningham, M., Everton, T., Hansen, A., Hopper, B., McIntyre, D., Oliver, C., Pell, T., Rouse, M. & Turner, P. (2007) *The Status of Teachers and the Teaching Profession in England: Views from Inside and Outside the Profession.* Evidence base for the Final Report of the Teacher Status Project. Nottingham: Department for Education and Science Publications. (Research Report RR831B).

Harris, K. J., Harvey, P., Harris, R. B. & Cast, M. (2013) An Investigation of Abusive Supervision, Vicarious Abusive Supervision, and Their Joint Impacts. *The Journal of Social Psychology*. 153(1). p.38–50.

Hauge, L. J., Einarsen, S., Knardahl, S., Lau, B., Notelaers, G. & Skogstad, A. (2011) Leadership and role stressors as departmental level predictors of workplace bullying. *International Journal of Stress Management*. 18(4). p.305–323.

Hauge, L. J., Skogstad, A. & Einarsen, S. (2007) Relationships between stressful work environments and bullying: Results of a large representative study. *Work & Stress*. 21(3). p.220–242.

Health and Safety Executive. (n.d.) What are the Management Standards for work related stress? [Online] Available from: http://www.hse.gov.uk/stress/standards/. [Accessed: January 29, 2014].

Hershcovis, M. S., Turner, N., Barling, J., Arnold, K. A., Dupré, K. E., Inness, M. & Sivanathan, N. (2007) Predicting workplace aggression: A meta-analysis. *Journal of Applied Psychology*. 92(1). p.228–238.

Higham, R. & Earley, P. (2013) School Autonomy and Government Control: School Leaders' Views on a Changing Policy Landscape in England. *Educational Management, Administration & Leadership*. 41(6). p.701–717.

Hoel, H. (2013) Workplace Bullying in United Kingdom. In JILPT Seminar on Workplace Bullying and Harassment. *Workplace Bullying and Harassment*. Tokyo: The Japan Institute for Labour Policy and Training (JILPT). (Report No. 12).

Hoel, H. & Cooper, C.L. (2000) *Destructive Conflict and Bullying at Work*. Manchester: Manchester School of Management, UMIST.

Hoel, H. & Cooper, C. (2001) Origins of bullying: theoretical frameworks for explaining workplace bullying. In Tehrani, N. (ed.). *Building a Culture of Respect: Managing Bullying at Work*. London: Taylor & Francis.

Hoel, H., Cooper, C. L. & Faragher, B. (2001) The experience of bullying in Great Britain: The impact of organizational status. *European Journal of Work and Organizational Psychology*. 10(4). p.443–465.

Hoel, H. & Giga, S. I. (2006) *Destructive Interpersonal Conflict in the Workplace: The Effectiveness of Management Interventions*.

Manchester Business School: The University of Manchester and British Occupational Health Research Foundation (BOHRF).

Hoel, H., Glasø, L., Hetland, J., Cooper, C. L. & Einarsen, S. (2010) Leadership Styles as Predictors of Self-reported and Observed Workplace Bullying. *British Journal of Management*. 21. p.453-468.

Hoel, H., Rayner, C. & Cooper, C.L. (1999) Workplace bullying. In Cooper, C. L. & Robertson, I. T. (eds.). *International review of industrial and organizational psychology*. Chichester: John Wiley & Sons.

Hogh, A., Hoel, H. & Carneiro, I. G. (2011) Bullying and employee turnover among healthcare workers: a three-wave prospective study. *Journal of Nursing Management*. 19(6). p.742–751.

Howard, M. L. (2012) *Headteacher Stress, Coping Strategies And Supports: Implications For An Emotional Health And Well-Being Programme* (Ed.D. Thesis). Manchester: Manchester University. [Online] Available from: http://ethos.bl.uk/OrderDetails. do?uin=uk.bl.ethos.632156.

Hubert, A. B. & van Veldhoven, M. (2001) Risk sectors for undesirable behaviour and mobbing. *European Journal of Work and Organizational Psychology*. 10(4). p.415–424.

Humphreys K. (1994) My Ball, Your Game: dilemmas in self-regulation according to the Ofsted criteria. *British Journal of In-Service Education*. 20(2). p.181-193.

Illing, J. C., Carter, M., Thompson, N. J., Crampton, P. E. S., Morrow, G. M., Howse, J. H. & Burford, B. C. (2013) *Evidence synthesis on the occurrence, causes, consequences, prevention and management of bullying and harassing behaviours to inform decision making in the NHS*. Durham Research Online (Project Report). London: HMSO.

Illingworth, J. (2010) *Reign of Terror: Links between school management (leadership), teacher stress and teacher mental health. An investigation and commentary*. [Online] March. Available from: www.teachermentalhealth.org.uk.

Irish National Teachers' Organization (INTO). (2000) *Staff Relations: A Report on Adult Bullying in Schools*. Dublin: Irish National Teachers' Organization. [Online] Available from: http://www.into.ie.

James, C., Brammer, S., Connolly, M., Spicer, D. E., James, J. & Jones, J. (2013) *The Chair of the School Governing Body in England: Roles, Relationships and Responsibilities.* CfBT Education Trust. [Online] Available from: http://cdn.cfbt.com/~/media/cfbtcorporate/files/research/2013/r-the-chair-of-the-school-governing-body-2013.pdf.

Jóhannsdóttir, H. L. & Ólafsson, R. F. (2004) Coping with bullying in the workplace: the effect of gender, age and type of bullying. *British Journal of Guidance & Counselling.* 32(3). p.319–333.

Karasek R. A. (1979) Job demands, job decision latitude, and mental strain: Implications for job redesign. *Administrative Science Quarterly.* 24(2). p.285–308.

Karasek, R.A. & Theorell, T. (1990) *Healthy work: stress, productivity, and the reconstruction of working life.* New York: Basic Books.

Keashly, L. & Jagatic, K. (2003) By any other name: American perspectives on workplace bullying. In Einarsen, S., Hoel, H., Zapf, D. & C. Cooper (eds.). *Bullying and emotional abuse in the workplace: International perspectives in research and practice.* London: Taylor and Francis.

Korkmaz, M. (2007) The Effects of Leadership Styles on Organizational Health. *Educational Research Quarterly.* 30(3). p.23–55.

Krasikova, D. V., Green, S. G. & LeBreton, J. M. (2013) Destructive Leadership: A Theoretical Review, Integration, and Future Research Agenda. *Journal of Management.* 39(5). p.1308–1338.

Lawton, D. (1973) *Social Change, Educational theory and Curriculum Planning.* London: University of London Press.

Lee, D. (2000) An analysis of workplace bullying in the UK. *Personnel Review.* 29(5). p.593–610.

Lehto A.M. & Pärnänen, A. (2007) *Violence, bullying and harassment in the workplace.* European Foundation for the Improvement of Living and Working Conditions. [Online] Available from: http://www.eurofound.europa.eu/observatories/eurwork/comparative-information/violence-bullying-and-harassment-in-the-workplace.

Leithwood, K. & Jantzi, D. (2006) Transformational school leadership for large-scale reform: Effects on students, teachers, and their classroom practices. *School Effectiveness and School Improvement.* 17(2). p.201–227.

Leithwood, K., Jantzi, D. & Steinbach, R. (eds.) (1999) *Changing Leadership for Changing Times.* Buckingham: Open University Press.

Lewis, D. (2004) Bullying at work: the impact of shame among university and college lecturers. *British Journal of Guidance & Counselling.* 32(3). p.281–299.

Lewis, D. & Gunn, R. (2007) Workplace bullying in the public sector: understanding the racial dimension. *Public Administration.* 85(3). p.641–665.

Leymann, H. (1996) The content and development of mobbing at work. *European Journal of Work and Organizational Psychology.* 5(2). p.165–184.

Leymann, H. & Gustafsson, A. (1996) Mobbing at work and the development of post-traumatic stress disorders. *European Journal of Work and Organizational Psychology.* 5(2). p.251–275.

Liefooghe, A.P.D. & Mackenzie Davey, K. (2001) Accounts of workplace bullying: the role of the organization. *European Journal of Work and Organizational Psychology.* 10(4). P.375-392.

Lindahl, R. A. (2007) Why is leading school improvement such a difficult process? *School Leadership & Management.* 27(4). p.319–332.

Lutgen-Sandvik, P. (2006) Take This Job and… : Quitting and Other Forms of Resistance to Workplace Bullying. *Communication Monographs.* 73(4). p.406–433.

MacBeath, J. (2011) No lack of principles: leadership development in England and Scotland. *School Leadership & Management.* 31(2). p.105–121.

MacBeath, J., Galton, M., (2008) Pressure and Professionalism: the impact of recent and present government policies on the working lives of teachers. ICSEI 21st International Congress for School Effectiveness and Improvement. Auckland, New Zealand. 6-9th January. [Online]. Available from: http://www.pbs.kau.se/pdf/ MacBeathGalton_icsei08.pdf.

MacBeath, J., O'Brien, J. & Gronn, P. (2012) Drowning or waving?

Coping strategies among Scottish head teachers. *School Leadership & Management.* 32(5). p.421–437.

Matthiesen, S. B. & Einarsen, S. (2001) MMPI-2 configurations among victims of bullying at work and organisational psychology. *European Journal of Work.* 10(4). p.467-484.

Matthiesen, S. & Einarsen, S. (2007) Perpetrators and targets of bullying at work: role stress and individual differences. *Violence and Victims.* 22(6). p.735–753.

McCormack, D., Casimir, G., Djurkovic, N. & Yang, L. (2009) Workplace Bullying and Intention to Leave Among Schoolteachers in China: The Mediating Effect of Affective Commitment. *Journal of Applied Social Psychology.* 39(9). p.2106–2127.

McGrath, D. L. (2010) The Abuse of Formal and Informal Power: Workplace Bullying as a Dichotomous Construct. *In 2nd Global Conference, Bullying and The Abuse of Power: From the Playground to International Relations.* [Online] p.1–9. Available from: http://www.inter-disciplinary.net/wp-content/uploads/2010/11/DLMcGrathPaper.pdf.

McMahon, A. (2001) Fair Furlong Primary School. In Maden, M. (ed.). *Success Against the Odds – Five Years On: Revisiting effective schools in disadvantaged areas.* London: Routledge Falmer.

Mind (2015) *How to manage stress.* Mind (National Association for Mental Health). [Online].Available from:
http://www.mind.org.uk/information-support/tips-for-everyday-living/stress/signs-of-stress.aspx#.VkoR2b_OtI4.

Morrell, G., Tennant, R., Kotecha, M., Newmark, T. & O'Connor, W. (2010) *Factors contributing to the referral and non-referral of incompetence cases to the GTC.* Prepared by The National Centre for Social Research for the General Teaching Council for England and the Department for Children, Schools and Families. [Online] January. Available from: http://217.35.77.12/research/england/education/GTC-10-01.pdf.

Mulholland, R., McKinlay, A. & Sproule, J. (2013) Teacher Interrupted: Work Stress, Strain, and Teaching Role. *SAGE Open.* July-September (09.2013). p.1-13.

NASUWT. (2011) *Teacher capability/competence: A review of the evidence.* NASUWT (11/04049). [Online]. Available from: http://www.nasuwt.org.uk/consum/groups/public/@press/documents/nas_download/nasuwt_008633.pdf. [Accessed: 3rd November 2015].

NASUWT. (2012) *Workplace bullying in schools and colleges.* NASUWT. (12/03017). [Online]. Available from: www.nasuwt.org.uk/consum/groups/public/.../nas.../nasuwt_009169.pdf. [Accessed: 3rd November 2015].

NASUWT. (2014) *NASUWT comments on the publication of the Teachers' Workload Diary Survey.* [Online]. Available from: http://www.politics.co.uk/opinion-formers/nasuwt-the-teachers-union/article/nasuwt-comments-on-the-publication-of-the-teachers-workload. [Accessed: 3rd November 2015].

National Governors' Association. (2015) *Being a school governor.* [Online} Available from: http://www.nga.org.uk/Be-a-Governor.aspx. [Accessed: 3rd November 2015].

Nielsen, M. B. (2013) Bullying in work groups: The impact of leadership. *Scandinavian Journal of Psychology.* 54(2). p.127–136.

Nielsen, M. B. & Einarsen, S. (2012) Outcomes of exposure to workplace bullying: A meta-analytic review. *Work & Stress.* 26(4). p.309–332.

Nielsen, M. B., Hetland, J., Matthiesen, S. B. & Einarsen, S. (2012) Longitudinal relationships between workplace bullying and psychological distress. *Scandinavian Journal of Work, Environment & Health.* 38(1). p.38–46.

Nielsen, M. B., Matthiesen, S. B. & Einarsen, S. (2010) The impact of methodological moderators on prevalence rates of workplace bullying: A meta-analysis. *Journal of Occupational and Organizational Psychology.* 83(4). p.955–979.

Nielsen, M. B., Skogstad, A., Matthiesen, S. B., Glasø, L., Aasland, M. S., Notelaers, G. & Einarsen, S. (2009) Prevalence of workplace bullying in Norway: Comparisons across time and estimation methods. *European Journal of Work and Organizational Psychology.* 18(1). p.81–101.

Notelaers, G., Baillien, E., De Witte, H., Einarsen, S. & Vermunt, J. K. (2013) Testing the strain hypothesis of the Demand Control

Model to explain severe bullying at work. *Economic and Industrial Democracy.* 34(1). p.69–87.

Notelaers, G., Vermunt, J. K., Baillien, E., Einarsen, S. & De Witte, H. (2011) Exploring risk groups workplace bullying with categorical data. *Industrial Health.* 49(1). p.73–88.

Nubling, M., Vomstein, M., Nubling, T. & Adiwidjaja, A. (2011) *European-Wide Survey on Teachers Work Related Stress – Assessment, Comparison and Evaluation of the Impact of Psychosocial Hazards on Teachers in their Workplace .* Freiburg, Germany: FFAS – Occupational and Social Medicine Research Centre Freiburg. (Final Report).

O'Connell, P. J., Calvert, E. & Watson, D. (2007) *Bullying in the Workplace: Survey Reports.* Ireland: The Economic and Social Research Institute. [Online] Available from: http://collection. europarchive.org/dnb/20070702132253/http://www.entemp.ie/publications/employment/2007/esrireportbullying.pdf.

O'Moore, M. (2000) *Bullying at Work in Ireland: A National Study.* Dublin: Anti Bullying Centre.

O'Moore, M., Seigne, E., McGuire, L. & Smith, M. (1998) Victims of workplace bullying in Ireland. *The Irish Journal of Psychology.* 19(2-3). p.345–357.

Office for Disability Issues. (2010) *Equality Act 2010 Guidance on matters to be taken into account in determining questions relating to the definition of disability.* HM Government. [Online] Available from: www.odi.gov.uk/equalityact.

Parent-Thirion, A., Macías, E. F., Hurley, J. & Vermeylen, G. (2007) *Fourth European Working Conditions Survey.* Dublin: European Foundation for the Improvement of Living and Working Conditions.

Phillips, S. J., Sen, D. & McNamee, R. (2008) Risk factors for work-related stress and health in head teachers. *Occupational Medicine.* 58(8). p.584–586.

Phillips, S., Sen, D. & McNamee, R. (2007) Prevalence and causes of self-reported work-related stress in head teachers. *Occupational Medicine.* 57(5). p.367–376.

Price Waterhouse Coopers, L. L. P. (2007) *Independent study into school leadership.* Nottingham: Department for Education and Skills. (No.

RR818A). [Online] Available from: http://www.cfbt.com/lincolnshire/ pdf/latest%20summary%20of%20pcw%20Jan%2007.pdf.

Quine, L. (2001) Workplace Bullying in Nurses. *Journal of Health Psychology.* 6(1). p.73–84.

Rayner, C. & Hoel, H. (1997) A Summary Review of Literature Relating to Workplace Bullying. *Journal of Community & Applied Social Psychology.* 7(3). p.181–91.

Rayner, C., Hoel, H. & Cooper, C.L. (2002) *Workplace Bullying: What we know, who is to blame and what can we do?* London: Taylor and Francis.

Riley, D., Duncan, D. J. & Edwards, J. (2011) Staff bullying in Australian schools. *Journal of Educational Administration.* 49(1). p.7–30.

Riley, D., Duncan, D. J. & Edwards, J. S. (2009) *Investigation of staff bullying in Australian schools: executive summary.* [Online] Available from: http://www.schoolbullies.org.au/ InvestigationOfStaffBullying_ExecSummary.pdf.

Robbins, S. (2013) Educational leadership programmes in the UK: Who cares about the school leader? *Management in Education.* 27(2). p.50–55.

Roscigno, V. J., Hodson, R. & Lopez, S. H. (2009) Workplace incivilities: the role of interest conflicts, social closure and organizational chaos. *Work, Employment & Society.* 23(4). p.747–773.

Roscigno, V. J., Lopez, S. H. & Hodson, R. (2009) Supervisory bullying, status inequalities and organizational context. *Social Forces.* 87(3). p.1561–1589.

Rothi, D., Leavey, G. & Loewenthal, K. (2010) *Teachers' mental health: a study exploring the experiences of teachers with work-related stress and mental health problems.* NASUWT. [Online] Available from: http://www.thedigitalpublisher.co.uk/mhealthreport2010.

Russo, A., Milić, R., Knežević, B., Mulić, R. & Mustajbegović, J. (2008) Harassment in Workplace Among School Teachers: Development of Survey. *Croatian Medical Journal.* 49(4). p.545–552.

Salin, D. (2001) Prevalence and forms of bullying among business professionals: A comparison of two different strategies for measuring bullying. *European Journal of Work and Organisational Psychology.* 10(4). p.425-441.

Salin, D. (2003) Ways of Explaining Workplace Bullying: A Review of Enabling, Motivating and Precipitating Structures and Processes in the Work Environment. *Human Relations.* 56(10). p.1213–1232.

Salin, D. & Hoel, H. (2011) Organisational causes of workplace bullying. In Einarsen, S., Hoel, H., Zapf, D. & Cooper, C. (eds.). *Bullying and Harassment in the Workplace: Developments in Theory, Research, and Practice.* 2nd Edition. Florida: CRC Press, Taylor and Francis Group.

Schyns, B. & Schilling, J. (2013) How bad are the effects of bad leaders? A meta-analysis of destructive leadership and its outcomes. *The Leadership Quarterly.* 24(1). p.138–158.

Seymour, L. & Grove, B. (2005) *Workplace interventions for people with common mental health problems.* London: British Occupational Health Research Foundation.

Sibieta, L. (2015)*The distribution of school funding and inputs in England:1993-2013.* London: The Institute for Fiscal Studies (IFS). [Online] Available from: http://www.ifs.org.uk/publications/7645.

Skogstad, A., Einarsen, S., Torsheim, T., Aasland, M. S. & Hetland, H. (2007). The destructiveness of laissez-faire leadership behaviour. *Journal of Occupational Health Psychology,* 12(1), 80–92.

Skogstad, A., Matthiesen, S. B. & Einarsen, S. (2007a) Organizational changes: a precursor of bullying at work? *International Journal of Organization Theory and Behavior.* 10(1). p.58-94.

Smith, P. & Bell, L. (2011) Transactional and transformational leadership in schools in challenging circumstances: a policy paradox. *Management in Education.* 25(2). p.58–61.

Strandmark, M. K. & Hallberg, L. R. M. (2007) The origin of workplace bullying: experiences from the perspective of bully victims in the public service sector. *Journal of Nursing Management.* 15(3). p.332–341.

Tafvelin, S. (2013) *The Transformational Leadership Process: Antecedents, Mechanisms, and Outcomes in the Social Services.* [Online] Available from: http://www.diva-portal.org/smash/record.jsf?pid=diva2:640843.

Teacher Support Network (2008) *Bullying of teachers a massive and highly damaging problem.* [Online] Available from: http://

teachersupport.info/news/announcements/Bullying-of-teachers-a-massiveproblem.php.

Tepper, B. J. (2000) Consequences of Abusive Supervision. *Academy of Management Journal*. 43(2). p.178–190.

Thornton, M. & Bricheno, P. (2006) *Missing Men in Education*. Stoke-on-Trent: Trentham Books.

Trépanier, S.-G., Fernet, C. & Austin, S. (2013) Workplace bullying and psychological health at work: The mediating role of satisfaction of needs for autonomy, competence and relatedness. *Work & Stress*. 27(2). p.123–140.

Troman G. (2008) Primary teacher identity, commitment and career in performative school cultures. *British Educational Research Journal*. 34(5). p.619–633.

Troman, G. & Woods, P. (2001) *Primary Teachers' Stress*. London: Routledge Falmer.

Unison. (2015) *Preventing Work-Related Mental Health Conditions By Tackling Stress. Guidance for School Leaders*, from NUT, GMB, Unison and Unite. [Online].Available from: https://www.unison. org.uk/content/uploads/2015/03/TowebPreventing-mental-health-conditions-by-tackling-stress-at-work-Jan-15.doc2.pdf.

Van Dick, R. & Wagner, U. (2001) Stress and strain in teaching: A structural equation approach. *British Journal of Educational Psychology*. 71(2) p.243–259.

Vartia, M. (1996) The sources of bullying –psychological work environment and organizational climate. *European Journal of Work and Organizational Psychology*. 5(2). p.203–214.

Webb R. & Vulliamy G. (1996) A Deluge of Directives: conflict between collegiality and managerialism in the post-ERA primary school. *British Educational Research Journal*. 22(4). p.441-458.

Webb, R., Vulliamy, G., Sarja, A., Hämäläinen, S. & Poikonen, P. L. (2012) Rewards, changes and challenges in the role of primary headteachers/principals in England and Finland. *Education 3-13*. 40(2). p.145–158.

West, P., Mattel P. & Roberts, J. (2011) Accountability and Sanctions in English Schools. *British Journal of Educational Studies*. 59(1). p.41-62.

Wilkins, C. (2011) Professionalism and the post-performative teacher: new teachers reflect on autonomy and accountability in the English school system. *Professional Development in Education.* 37(3). p.389–409.

Woods, P. A., Woods, G. J. & Cowie, M. (2009) Tears, laughter, camaraderie: professional development for headteachers. *School Leadership & Management.* 29(3). p.253–275.

Zapf, D., Escartin, J., Einarsen, S., Hoel, H. & Vartia, M. (2011) Empirical findings on prevalence and risk groups of bullying in the workplace. In Einarsen, S., Hoel, H., Zapf, D. & Cooper, C. (eds.). *Bullying and Harassment in the Workplace: Developments in Theory, Research, and Practice.* 2nd Edition. Florida US: CRC Press, Taylor and Francis Group.

Zapf, D. (*1999*) Organisational, work group related and personal causes of mobbing/bullying at work. *International Journal of Manpower.* 12 (*1/2*). p.*70-85.*

Zapf, D. & Einarsen, S. (2011) Individual antecedents of bullying: victims and perpetrators. In Einarsen, S., Hoel, H., Zapf, D. & C. Cooper (eds.). *Bullying and Harassment in the Workplace: Developments in Theory, Research, and Practice.* 2nd Edition. Florida US: CRC Press, Taylor and Francis Group.

Zapf, D., Knorz, C. & Kulla, M. (1996) On the relationship between mobbing factors, and job content, social work environment, and health outcomes. *European Journal of Work and Organizational Psychology.* 5(2). p.215–237.

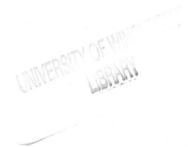